Practical Immunocytochemistry
in Diagnostic Cytology

Eugenio Leonardo • Ricardo H. Bardales

Practical Immunocytochemistry in Diagnostic Cytology

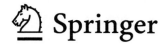

Eugenio Leonardo
First level Pathologist Doctor
San Lazzaro Hospital
Alba, Italy

Ricardo H. Bardales
Director Fine Needle Aspiration Service
Precision Pathology / Outpatient Pathology
Associates
Sacramento, CA
USA

ISBN 978-3-030-46658-9   ISBN 978-3-030-46656-5   (eBook)
https://doi.org/10.1007/978-3-030-46656-5

This Springer imprint is published by the registered company Springer Nature Switzerland AG
The registered company address is: Gewerbestrasse 11, 6330 Cham, Switzerland

My parents Waldetrudis and Ricardo, who patiently taught me the value of education
Angela, Angie, and Ricky for their constant encouragement, support, and tolerance
My mentors Abel Mejia, Benjamin Koziner, Leopold G. Koss, Klaus Schreiber, Norwin Becker, Michael W. Stanley, and John Abele
My Pathology residents and Cytology fellows

Ricardo H. Bardales, MD, FIAC, ECNU

My parents Maria Paola and Bruno for their love and guidance through life

Eugenio Leonardo, MD, PhD

Preface

An accurate and reliable diagnosis of neoplastic and non-neoplastic processes made in cyto-logic material harvested by minimally invasive procedures is always welcomed by treating physicians and patients. Cytologic diagnosis alone provides crucial information; however, immunocytochemistry (ICC) performed in the cytologic material obtained by exfoliative methods or fine-needle aspiration (FNA) gives additional information and complements the cytologic diagnosis. In fact, by combining appropriate antibodies it is possible to complement cellular aspects with molecular information and improve the accuracy of the cytologic diagno-sis to positively impact patient care.

The ICC should no longer be considered a "special staining" to be applied to histologic and cytologic samples; instead, it must be considered a diagnostic method that joins, with equal dignity, histo- and cyto-morphologic investigations to better define the nature of a mass. Therefore, ICC must be considered a "molecular stain" and sometimes a substitute for molecu-lar biology tests. ICC has become a routine activity applied to the diagnostic field and is now a necessary and, in some cases, indispensable method that allows the pathologist to clarify the real nature of cellular structures where cytomorphology alone has limitations. Despite existing similarities, there are critical differences between the immunostain performed on histologic and on cytologic samples. Understanding these differences is fundamental for the correct exe-cution and interpretation of ICC stains.

The purpose of this book is twofold: (1) To provide practical information for the appropriate handling and preparation of cytologic samples to reduce the risk of artifacts and avoid false positive or false negative results. Technical details, exclusively derived from our daily experi-ence, are included in the first chapter, while the last chapter deals with stain artifacts and pos-sible misinterpretations of immunostainings. (2) To provide a systematic description of the immunophenotypic and biomolecular characteristics that are present in benign and malignant cells useful for the practical solution of cytologic differential diagnoses. Only the morphologic-molecular structures of proven validation are reported.

In summary, this book provides an up-to-date judicious use of conventional and molecular ICC markers performed in cytologic samples to help in the diagnosis in a cost-effective man-ner. A cytologic differential diagnosis will be followed to construct a sequence/algorithm of ICC stains to provide appropriate, and in some cases personalized, therapy. All chapters include description of the cytomorphology of lesions/tumors followed by a practical ICC staining pat-tern. Cytologic samples include exfoliative cytology including serous effusions, FNA of super-ficial and deep-seated masses, and squash preparations from central nervous system tumors.

This book will be a valuable source of information for practicing pathologists, residents in pathology, cytopathology fellows, and cytotechnologists interested in acquiring knowledge on the role of ICC in cytopathology diagnosis.

Alba, Italy   Eugenio Leonardo, MD, PhD
Sacramento, CA, USA   Ricardo H. Bardales, MD, FIAC, ECNU

Acknowledgements

Our special thanks to the Pathology residents and fellows, who throughout the years have contributed with cases that always occupy special places in the library of our desks and most important our hearts. Also, we thank Mrs. Lorraine P. Coffey, Developmental Editor, and Richard Hruska, Senior Editor for Springer Nature for their constant support and patience. Last but not least, our special gratitude and admiration to Mrs. Elisabeth Lanzl, Senior Editor at the University of Chicago, for her undaunted effort to improve the English grammar and syntax of our manuscripts to transform them into readable documents.

Eugenio Leonardo, MD, PhD
Ricardo H. Bardales, MD, FIAC, ECNU

Contents

Immunocytochemistry: Technical Considerations Applied to Cytology

1.1 Collection and Transport of Cytologic Samples

Immunocytochemistry has become an important activity for the complete and accurate diagnosis of cytologic preparations. The outcome of the immunocytochemical method depends not only on good preservation of the cytomorphology but also on maintenance of the antigenic structures.

Four different methods can be used for the collection of a cytologic sample: (1) insertion of the biological sample into a transport medium, (2) placement of the cytologic material directly into a fixative solution, (3) collection of the material without addition of either transport solutions or fixatives, and (4) smearing of the sample directly onto a glass slide, without any kind of pre-treatment.

1. The transport medium of the cytologic sample must be a solution able to block the phenomenon of cellular self-digestion, preserving both the morphologic and the antigenic integrity of the cells. The best solutions for the transfer of cytologic material include culture medium or Michael's solution. However, if the material is to be processed without delay, cold physiologic solutions or buffered solutions with physiologic pH and molarity can also be used as transport media.

   Many commercially available transport liquids contain mixtures with different concentrations of polyethylene glycol and methyl alcohol. If the alcohol concentration is small, the subsequent immunostains can be carried out without problems, whereas if a solution is composed of a high quantity of methyl alcohol, isopropanol, or ethyl alcohol, commonly there is a change or denaturation of most antigens, with the result of a possible false immunocytochemical reaction.

2. Cytology samples can also be collected directly in fixative solutions. In our experience, a cold (4–6 °C) solution of neutral buffered formalin, diluted at 0.5–1%, allows opti-

mal cellular preservation, maintaining both the cytomorphologic features and the molecular integrity of the antigen. If the cells are fixed in suspension, they tend to maintain their three-dimensional configuration, because of the stiffness given to the cytoplasmic membrane by the solution. Therefore, blood elements will maintain their spheroidal or ovoid shape, whereas epithelial cells will tend to assume a flat configuration.

3. If the cytologic sample consists of a serous effusion, it can be collected in containers without transport medium and/or fixative solutions. However, it is then necessary to operate under sterile conditions with cold containers and to send the samples to the cytology laboratory as quickly as possible. Then, the cytologic sample must be processed immediately or within a short period of time, according to standardized laboratory procedures.

4. Another possibility is the rapid preparation of cytologic smears immediately after collection. The choice of whether or not to fix a cytologic smear depends on the type of cytologic procedure to be performed, because both ways are potentially compatible with the subsequent execution of immunostaining. However, it should be noted that fixation mainly preserves cellular morphologic characteristics. Rapid fixation of the cells after the preparation of the smear usually allows a better morphologic appearance than does air-drying, allowing a better preservation of different cellular and subcellular structures, favoring a better detail of the nuclear and cytoplasmic characteristics. Consequently, adequate treatment of the cytologic material is indispensable.

If the cytologic sample contains sufficient material, it is possible to use preparations by different methods, among which the cell block is an important one. However, if the cytologic sample has poor cellularity, it is necessary to choose a concentrating method for preparing the cytologic sample.

© Springer Nature Switzerland AG 2020
E. Leonardo, R. H. Bardales, *Practical Immunocytochemistry in Diagnostic Cytology*,
https://doi.org/10.1007/978-3-030-46656-5_1

1.2   Preparation of the Cytologic Sample

1.2.1   Smears

A cytologic smear is prepared by placement of a drop of the sample on a glass slide and then, by use of another slide, gentle but firm extension of the material is made so that the smear obtained is thin and homogeneously distributed along the major axis of the slide. The smear can then be used for immunocytochemical investigations according to the most appropriate technique for the predetermined purpose.

1.2.2   Imprints

Cytology by apposition of a tissue sample onto a glass slide "transforms" a histologic sample into a cytologic preparation. In fact, it uses the capacity of cells to adhere to the smooth surface of the glass slide. The technique is very simple: a fragment of the tissue is placed on a slide, with exerting of weak pressure, so that the cellular elements present on the surface of the tissue separate and adhere to the glass slide.

The imprint technique is used in specimens from superficial skin lesions and, in some surgical biopsies, for quick evaluation of the cell population. A typical example is the imprinting of excised lymph nodes, bone marrow biopsies, or small neurosurgical biopsies.

1.2.3   Cytospin

The cytospin technique is the method of choice when the cytologic sample consists of a small amount of fluid that contains a variable number of dispersed cells. A typical example is cerebrospinal fluid. The preparation is carried out with use of a special centrifuge in which a special holder containing the cytologic sample is placed. The subsequent centrifugation distributes the cells on the surface of a glass slide in a monolayer, which is usually circular, with a diameter of 4–8 mm.

1.3   Polycarbonate Membrane Filtration

In the case of liquid cytology samples with high cell dispersion, membrane filtration is a method that allows good recovery of cells. It is applied especially in urinary cytology. In practice, the cytologic sample is placed in a hollow cylinder (often a 50 ml device) which, at one end, connects a filter with a porous filtration membrane that usually has a circular shape with a diameter between 10 and 20 mm. The cells are stratified on the surface of the membrane and subsequently transferred onto a glass slide that had been cooled to improve the cell adhesiveness.

1.4   Liquid-Based Cytology

Liquid-based cytology is a technique that enables cells suspended in a liquid medium to be spread in a monolayer, so that a better morphologic assessment is possible. This includes the preparation and evaluation of cells collected by various methods (brushings, fine-needle aspiration) and placed in a preservative liquid, usually consisting of polyethylene glycol or methyl alcohol. This is then placed on a computerized instrument that operates cell dispersion, removing any mucus and any cellular debris that may be present, without modifying the morphology of the cells. Through a device that is controlled by a special microprocessor which checks the flow in the liquid phase, the cells are harvested while the percentage of the different cellular strains present is preserved and are ultimately distributed in the monolayer in a pre-established quantity (50,000–70,000 cells).

We must remember that the presence of ethyl alcohol and/or methanol can, in fact, modify the antigenic structure of some molecules.

1.5   Cell Block

The cell-block method may be performed simultaneously with or as an alternative to other cytologic preparations, with the goal of combining the advantages of cytology techniques with those of histopathology. In other words, a cytologic sample is transformed into a histologic one. Briefly, it is necessary first to concentrate the cells by centrifugation, followed by removal of the supernatant and the collection of cell sediment. The cells are then re-suspended in a fixative medium, usually 4–5% neutral buffered formalin, and left to fix, preferably at 4–6 °C, for 10–20 minutes. After further centrifugation, the cell sediment is dehydrated with a series of alcohols, clarified with diaphanizing solutions, embedded in paraffin, and cut with a microtome, similar to of what happens for histologic samples. The cell-block preparation of the cytologic sample increases the possibility of morphologic diagnoses, because it allows a better evaluation of the aggregated cell elements, limiting cell overlapping and reducing interference by the presence of red cells and cellular debris. Moreover, the inclusion in paraffin allows an optimal conservation of the sample and the possibility of carrying out subsequent immunohistochemical investigations with a large antibody panel.

The technical difficulty of collecting sediment is often reported for samples with poor cellularity. We can overcome this problem by pre-inclusion of the sample in agar, celloidin, or a fibrin clot. The "pre-inclusion systems" facilitate the collection of the entire sediment and prevent the loss of cells during the subsequent steps. The method that uses neutral agar involves coating of the cellular sediment with this substance immediately after fixation and before dehydrating of the sample. The method with celloidin involves the preparation of a celloidin solution, which is obtained by dissolving of 10 g of this substance in 100 ml. of a mixture composed of ethyl alcohol and ethyl ether. A tube is filled with this solution and then with chloroform, so that the celloidin film is hardened and excessive drying is prevented. Finally, the cytologic sample is suspended in 10% neutral buffered formalin, put in a test tube, and centrifuged at 1000 g/min for 10 minutes. The supernatant is discarded, the upper part of the film is eliminated, and the sediment is recovered. The procedure that involves the formation of the coagulum is performed by centrifuging of the cytologic sample, removal of the supernatant, and then addition of a few drops of plasma followed by a small amount of thrombin, to form a clot. This is then fixed and processed like a histologic sample.

1.6 Fixation and Dehydration of the Sample

In the preparation of the cytologic sample, with the exception of the cell-block method, a crucial point is to choose between the immediate fixation of the cells adhering to a glass slide or, on the contrary, dehydration of the cells before fixation. There are three different choices for fixing smears: (1) spraying the slide with a Cytospray solution (usually consisting of polyethylene glycol or methyl alcohol), (2) immersion of the slide in a 95% ethyl alcohol solution, or (3) allowing the smear to air-dry. The most common dehydrating method is to let the water "evaporate" by leaving the cytologic preparations in the air, at room temperature, for a few hours. That time can be reduced to 1–2 hours by use of a portable fan for air-drying of the smears.

In cases where there is a presumptive diagnosis of a hemolymphoproliferative disorder, smears, cytospins, and imprints provide an improved yield when they are first air-dried and then fixed. On the contrary, fixation before dehydration may be preferred for cytologic material harvested by fine-needle aspiration. It must still be born in mind that some fixatives can partially or irreversibly denature the antigens. The fixation must be carried out for an adequate time by use of a fixative that allows a good cytomorphology without causing antigen molecular alterations and with allowing the performance of useful immunocytochemical investigations.

In our laboratory, the use of solutions (v/v) of acetone and chloroform (1:1), or, better, of acetone and methanol (1:1), at 4–6 °C for 10–15 minutes, renders a suitable cytomorphology that is adequate for cytologic interpretation and suitable for immunostaining using most antibodies.

For cytologic air-dried preparations or those treated with polyethylene glycol spray only (without methanol), we routinely use a fixation solution consisting of 0.1% neutral saline formalin for 30 minutes at room temperature. This solution is obtained by addition of 0.25 ml of paraformaldehyde (formalin 37%) to 100 ml of phosphate buffer (PBS), 0.1 M and pH 7.4. Alternatively, good results can be obtained with the use of 10% neutral buffered formalin for 10–15 minutes at room temperature or for 30 minutes at 4–6 °C. Another possibility is the fixation of cytologic preparations for 1–2 hours at room temperature with a solution consisting of 50 ml of absolute ethyl alcohol, 5 ml of 40% polyethylene glycol, 5 ml of paraformaldehyde, and 40 ml of distilled water.

1.7 Preservation of Cytologic Preparations for Immunocytochemical Reactions

Air-dried smears, even if they have been fixed with alcohol before drying, will probably undergo antigen deterioration, unless they have been frozen and stored at −80 °C. Also, formalin-fixed smears should be stored at low temperature. Their use for immunostaining must be preceded by rehydration in normal saline for at least 5 minutes.

There are two simple methods for preserving the morphology and conserving the antigenicity of cytologic samples: (1) the first method applies to smears, imprints, or cytospins. After rapid fixation (30–60 sec) in 95° ethyl alcohol and without allowing the cytologic preparation to dry, the cells adhering to the slide are coated with a 10% polyethylene glycol solution in 10% methanol, left to dry at room temperature, and then stored at a low temperature. The polyethylene glycol forms a thin film on the cytologic preparation and therefore protects the antigens and does not alter the cellular morphology. The film is removed before the immunostaining procedure by washing of the slide with an alcohol solution. Subsequently, the cytologic sample must be fixed with the same chosen fixative solution. (2) The second possibility is to place the cellular sample directly into a polyethylene glycol/10% methanol solution. In this solution, the cytologic material can be stored at room temperature for approximately 30 days, and it can be used for DNA extraction, RNA, genetic studies, and in situ hybridization in addition to immunocytochemistry.

1.8 Antigen Retrieval

The restoration of antigenicity, or reactivation, is always a necessary procedure for cell blocks when the material has been fixed in formalin and when the same procedures are used as those for histologic preparations. It is also essential to perform reactivation treatments if the cells of smears and/or of imprints have undergone aldehyde fixation. The smears and the analogous cytologic preparations fixed in formalin can be subjected to a reactivation intervention in citrate buffer by use of a microwave oven and performance of two cycles of heating for 3 minutes each with powers of 350–450 Watts.

The method which we use to restore antigenicity of cytologic samples makes use of a solution of citric acid at pH 7 with NaOH and the addition of 0.1% of a non-ionic surfactant in a high-temperature bain-marie (95–96 °C) for 5 minutes. The recovery of epitopes in cytologic preparations not fixed with solutions containing aldehydes, theoretically, should be without changes of the antigenic reaction. However, we have observed that a mild antigenic reactivation treatment improves the yield of immunostaining for certain antigens, sometimes in an unpredictable way. This phenomenon, also referred to by other centers of immunohistochemistry, still appears today without having a logical interpretation. In our experience, the best results for smear or imprint preparations are obtained in slides that are air-dried prior to alcohol fixation, whereas we observed a lower response for cells fixed with alcoholic solutions immediately after preparation.

1.9 Immunostaining of Cytologic Preparations

There are many methods for immunostaining of cytologic samples. The most-used method is the indirect two-step enzymatic procedure. Briefly, after antigen retrieval, the primary antibody, monoclonal or polyclonal, is placed on the cytologic preparation, and it binds the retrieved antigen if present and unchanged. The secondary antibody is directed against the immunoglobulin which constitutes the primary antibody and therefore binds to this one. The secondary antibody conveys enzymatic tracer molecules (peroxidase or alkaline phosphatase) through chemical bonds with polymers. The enzymatic tracer reacts with its substrate, a chromogen which precipitates on the site of the antigen/antibody reaction. The chromogen can therefore be visualized under light microscopy. Usually, a nuclear contrast coloring counterstain is also performed.

Because cells may contain enzymes similar to those used as tracers, some procedures must be performed which block the endogenous enzymes and prevent their reaction in the phase of visualization of the enzymatic tracer combined with the antibody. The endogenous enzyme blockage is performed before the incubation of the primary antibody, with use of an excess of the enzymatic substrate

(hydrogen peroxide in the case of peroxidase and levamisole in the case of alkaline phosphatase).

Sometimes, some receptors present on the cells can bind the applied antibodies in a non-specific way through electric charge reactions or hydrophobic bonds. Such antibodies bound in a non-specific way will react in the same way as do the specific ones and give a false-positive result. Non-specific reactions may be blocked by use of nonimmune serum of the same species as that of the secondary antibody, prior to the application of the primary antibody.

There is also the possibility that the primary antibody binds specifically to tissue antigens that share the same amino acid sequences, or a particular molecular configuration, with the investigated antigen (cross-reactions). If the characteristics of the primary antibody used are known, false interpretations of the results are reduced. However, any unexpected results should be studied with this possibility in mind.

Primary antibodies may be supplied "ready to use" or as a concentrate. In our laboratory, we prefer to use antibodies acquired in concentrated form, which we dilute before use. Monoclonal antibodies usually are used in a concentration of 1–3 µg/ml. However, it is good to try out the best dilution to be used. If positive control cytology preparations are not available, tests may be performed on appropriate paraffin-embedded tissue sections, and the optimal dilution chosen will be suitable for cytologic preparations. In our laboratory, we use a phosphate buffer solution of 0.01 M at pH 7.4, containing 0.1% bovine serum albumin (BSA) and 0.1% sodium azide as a preservative. The BSA acts as an inert protein that, by binding on the walls of the vial, allows the antibody molecules to be kept free in the solution. The primary antibodies diluted in this solution can be stored at 4 °C for a few days. In our laboratory, we usually incubate the sample with the primary antibody solution for 30 minutes at room temperature. The detection system (the secondary antibody carrying the enzymatic tracer) is allowed to react for about 30 minutes at room temperature.

It is also necessary to use positive and negative controls for each immunocytochemical reaction that is carried out. Positive controls consist of tissue sections that definitely contain the antigen. We use material coming from surgical excisions or cell blocks, rather than autopsy tissue samples, to avoid possible interference with immunostaining due to possible autolysis phenomena. We prefer to use multiblock or tissue array sections, which simultaneously contain different expressions of the antigen until it is completely absent. This system allows one to verify at the same time whether the immunocytochemical reaction has been carried out correctly (positive control) in the absence of non-specific bonds (negative control).

1.10 Automated Systems for Immunocytochemical Reactions

Currently, many laboratories use automatic and semiautomatic systems for immunohistochemical diagnostic routines.

1.11 Automatic Immunostainer Systems

These can be used only for cell-block cytology. This is due to the fact that current immunostainers have software with staining procedures that cannot be modified by the user, except partially for some parameters, such as time and incubation temperature, within ranges defined by the manufacturer. Another characteristic of the current instruments is that they are able to work exclusively with specific dedicated reagents, usually pre-diluted, and supplied by the manufacturer/distributor of the appliance in particular devices to be connected to the mechanical part of the instrument. These features allow automated immunostaining only for cell-block sections, as they are similar to histologic sections, whereas the immunostaining of smears, imprints, or cytospins is not possible, because they require times and temperatures that are lower than those set by the instrument.

1.12 Semiautomatic Systems

These systems allow one to modify any of the parameters proposed in the immunostaining procedure and even the creation, via software, of one's own laboratory-specific immunostaining protocols. Semiautomatic immunostainers allow the use of non-dedicated reagents, which can also be acquired from sources other than the manufacturer/distributor of the instrument and allow the user to work with diluted reagents according to his/her own needs and standardizations. This is advantageous not only in terms of the quality of the immune reactions but also in considerable cost containment.

Suggested Reading

Biesterfeld S, et al. Analysis of the reliability of manual and automated immunohistochemical staining procedures. A pilot study. Anal Quant Cytol Histol. 2003;25:90.

Dabbs DJ, et al. Immunochytochemistry on the ThinPrep processor. Diagn Cytopathol. 1997;17:388.

Dinges HP, et al. Immunocytochemistry in cytology: comparative evaluation of different tecniques. Quant Cytol Histol. 1989;11:22.

Fetsch PA, Abati A. Immunocytochemistry in effusion cytology: a contemporary review. Cancer (Cancer Cytopathol). 2001;93:293.

Fetsch PA, et al. Comparison of three commonly used cytologic preparations in effusion immunocytochemistry. Diagn Cytopathol. 2002;26:61.

Hunt JL, et al. Immunohistochemical analysis of gel-transferred cells in cytologic preparations following smear division. Diagn Cytopathol. 1998;18:377.

Kaplan MA, et al. Evaluation of CytoLyt and PreservCyt as preservatives for immunocytochemistry for cytokeratin in fine needle aspiration. Appl Immunohistochem. 1998;6:23.

Leong ASY. Immunostaining of cytologic specimens. Am J Clin Pathol. 1996;39:140.

Leung SW, Bedard YC. Immunocytochemical staining on ThinPrep processed smears. Mod Pathol. 1996;9:301.

O'Leary TJ. Cytopathology. In: Advanced diagnostic methods in pathology. Principles, practice, and protocols. Philadelphia: Saunders Company; 2003.

Osborn M, Domagala W. Immunocytochemistry. In: Bibbo M, editor. Comprehensive cytopathology. second ed. Philadelphia: W.B. Saunders Company; 1997.

Polak JM, Van Noorden S, editors. Immunocytochemistry: modern methods and applications. second ed. Bristol: Wright PSG; 1986.

Sherman ME, et al. Immunostaining of small cytologic specimens. Facilitation with cell transfer. Acta Cytol. 1994;38:18.

Shield PW, et al. Immunocytochemical staining of cytologic specimens: how helpful is it? Am J Clin Pathol. 1996;105:157.

Stoward PJ. Fixation in histochemistry. London: Chapman and Hall Eds; 1973.

Whinney WH, et al. Automated immunochemistry. Clin Pathol. 1990;43:591.

2.1 Normal Mesothelial Cells

Normal mesothelial cells can appear single or multinucleated, can be of varying sizes, and are generally larger than monocytes. In contrast to monocytes, they have more abundant cytoplasm, round and not folded nuclei, and an unapparent nucleolus (Fig. 2.1). Co-expression of CK5 (Fig. 2.2), CK6, CK7, CK8, CK14, CK 17, CK18, CK 19, calretinin (Fig. 2.3), WT-1 (Fig. 2.4), podoplanin (Fig. 2.5), vimentin, and BAP-1 (Fig. 2.6) is observed in mesothelial cells. Normal mesothelial cells express desmin (Fig. 2.7), but not EMA.

2.2 Reactive Mesothelial Cells

Serous inflammatory effusions caused by infectious, inflammatory, or reactive processes contain reactive mesothelial cells, histiocytes, neutrophils, eosinophils, and lymphocytes in variable numbers and proportions.

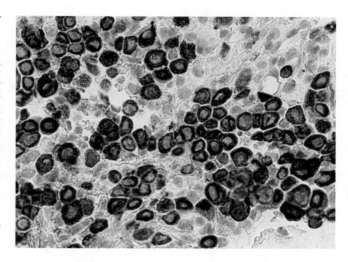

Fig. 2.2 Normal mesothelial cells. CK5 immunostain (high magnification)

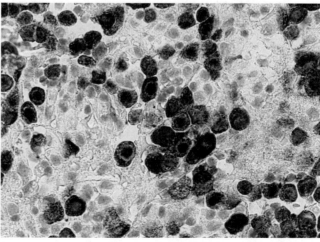

Fig. 2.3 Normal mesothelial cells. Calretinin immunostain (high magnification)

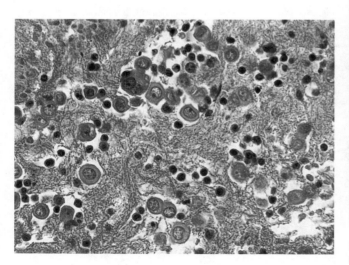

Fig. 2.1 Normal mesothelial cells. Cell block. H&E (high magnification)

© Springer Nature Switzerland AG 2020
E. Leonardo, R. H. Bardales, *Practical Immunocytochemistry in Diagnostic Cytology*,
https://doi.org/10.1007/978-3-030-46656-5_2

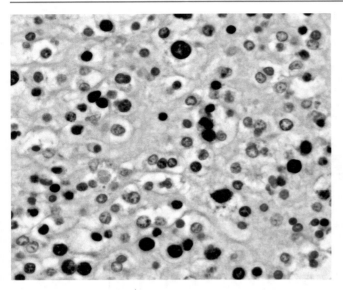

Fig. 2.4 Normal mesothelial cells. WT-1 immunostain (high magnification)

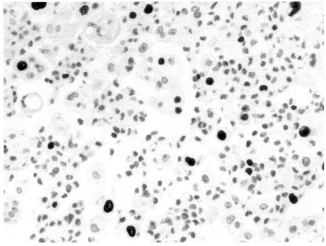

Fig. 2.6 Normal mesothelial cells. BAP—1 immunostain (high magnification)

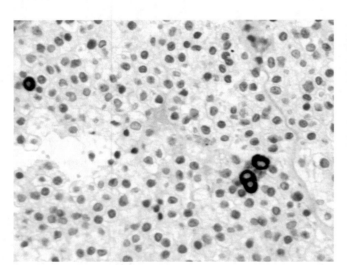

Fig. 2.5 Normal mesothelial cells. Podoplanin immunostain (high magnification)

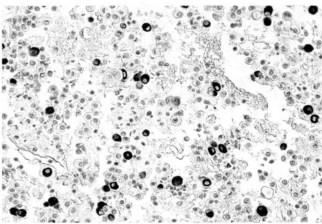

Fig. 2.7 Normal mesothelial cells. Desmin immunostain (high magnification)

Reactive mesothelial cells can be found in viral, bacterial, mycobacterial, fungal, and parasitic infectious conditions, as well as in reactive serous effusions of various etiologies, such as congestive heart failure, pulmonary embolism, myocardial infarction, cirrhosis, nephrotic syndrome, autoimmune diseases, pancreatitis, and trauma.

Mesothelial cells can be sparse or numerous, usually dispersed or gathered in small clusters. They have abundant cytoplasm and well-defined nuclei (Fig. 2.8). Sometimes they show binucleation or multinucleation (Fig. 2.9), whereas cytoplasmic vacuoles are less common.

Reactive mesothelial cells have the same immunophenotype as do normal mesothelial cells (Figs. 2.10, 2.11, and 2.12).

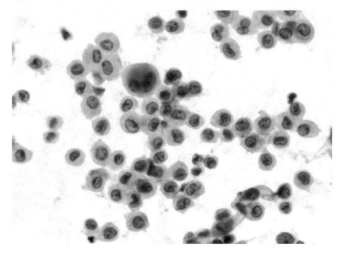

Fig. 2.8 Reactive mesothelial cells. Papanicolaou stain (high magnification)

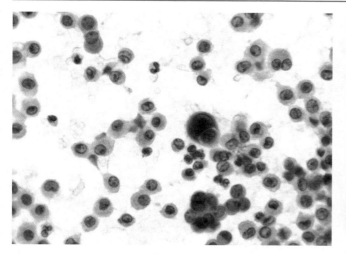

Fig. 2.9 Reactive mesothelial cells. Papanicolaou stain (high magnification)

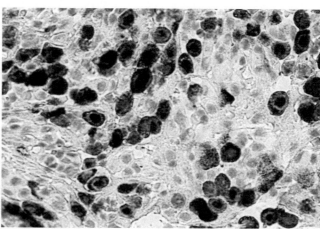

Fig. 2.12 Reactive mesothelial cells. WT-1 immunostain (high magnification)

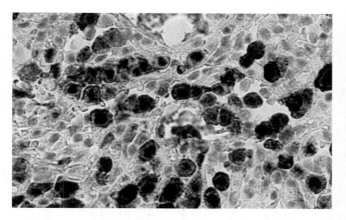

Fig. 2.10 Reactive mesothelial cells. Calretinin immunostain (high magnification)

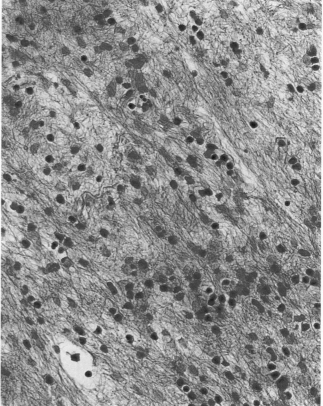

Fig. 2.13 Lymphocytic effusion. H&E (high magnification)

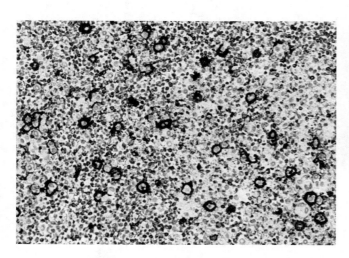

Fig. 2.11 Reactive mesothelial cells. Podoplanin immunostain (high magnification)

The cytologic interpretation of an acute inflammatory serous effusion usually does not show diagnostic difficulties, and immunocytochemistry is unnecessary.

Serous effusion with numerous lymphocytes (Fig. 2.13) may be difficult to differentiate from secondary involvement

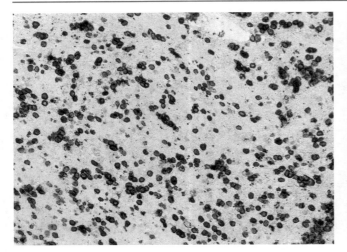

Fig. 2.14 Lymphocytic effusion. CD3 immunostain (high magnification)

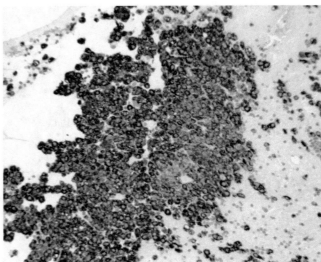

Fig. 2.16 Histiocytic effusion. H&E (high magnification)

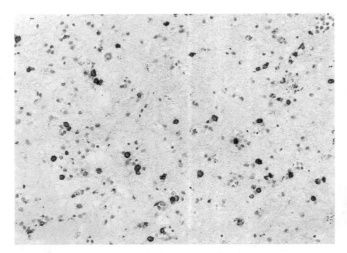

Fig. 2.15 Lymphocytic effusion. CD20 immunostain (high magnification)

Fig. 2.17 Histiocytic effusion. CD68 immunostain (medium magnification)

by small-cell lymphoma without help of ancillary tests. The absence of monoclonal lymphocytes directs the diagnosis toward an inflammatory condition (Figs. 2.14 and 2.15), whereas the finding of a monoclonal population is consistent with the presence of lymphoma.

The presence of numerous histiocytes (Fig. 2.16) can sometimes simulate a primary mesothelial neoplasm. Positive immunostaining for histiocytic markers such as CD68 (Fig. 2.17) or CD163 (Fig. 2.18), among others, allows one to recognize the inflammatory nature of a serous effusion.

2.3　Mesothelial Hyperplasia

This process is characterized by a reactive proliferation of the mesothelium that is arranged in multiple layers, sometimes showing a pseudopapillary (Fig. 2.19) or pseudonodular

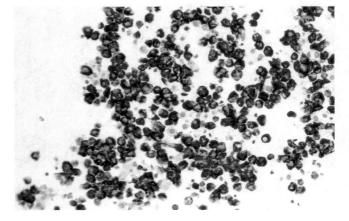

Fig. 2.18 Histiocytic effusion. CD163 immunostain (high magnification)

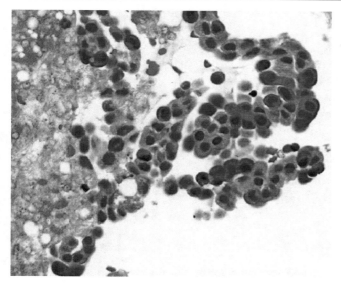

Fig. 2.19 Pseudopapillary hyperplasia. H&E (medium magnification)

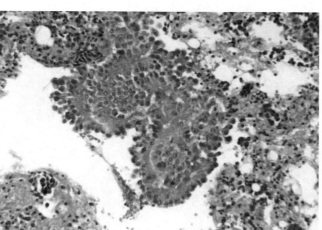

Fig. 2.20 Pseudonodular hyperplasia. H&E (high magnification)

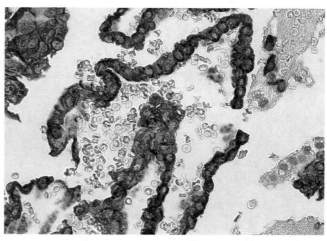

Fig. 2.21 Mesothelial hyperplasia. CK5 immunostain (high magnification)

Fig. 2.22 Mesothelial hyperplasia. CK7 immunostain (high magnification)

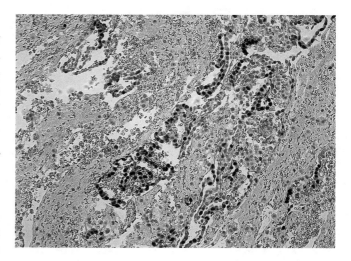

Fig. 2.23 Mesothelial hyperplasia. Calretinin immunostain (medium magnification)

architecture (Fig. 2.20). The mesothelial cells show positivity for CK5 (Fig. 2.21), CK6, CK7 (Fig. 2.22), CK8, CK14, CK17, CK18, CK19, HBME-1, HMFG, calretinin (Fig. 2.23), podoplanin (Fig. 2.24), WT-1 (Fig. 2.25), BAP-1 (Fig. 2.26), desmin (Fig. 2.27), membrane EMA (Fig. 2.28), and vimentin, whereas GLUT-1, IMP-3, and claudin are negative.

2.4 Primary Mesothelial Tumors

2.4.1 Mesothelioma

Epithelioid mesotheliomas and the epithelioid component of biphasic mesotheliomas are commonly associated with a serous effusion, whereas sarcomatous cells of the biphasic mesothelioma and cells of sarcomatous or desmoplas-

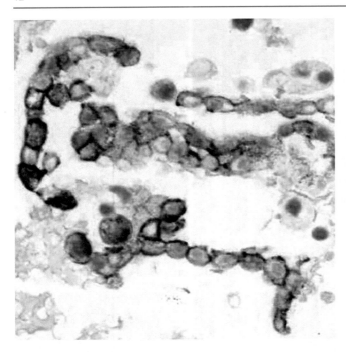

Fig. 2.24 Mesothelial hyperplasia. Podoplanin immunostain (high magnification)

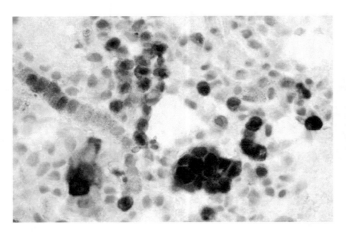

Fig. 2.25 Mesothelial hyperplasia. WT-1 immunostain (high magnification)

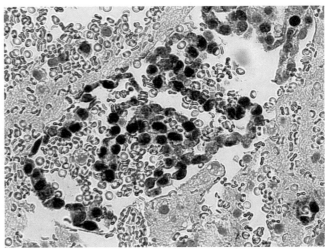

Fig. 2.26 Mesothelial hyperplasia. BAP-1 immunostain (high magnification)

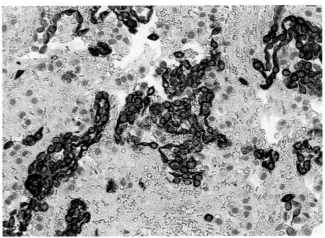

Fig. 2.27 Mesothelial hyperplasia. Desmin immunostain (high magnification)

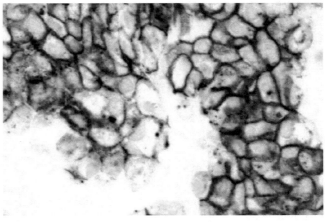

Fig. 2.28 Mesothelial hyperplasia. EMA immunostain (high magnification)

tic mesothelioma usually do not spontaneously exfoliate into associated effusions.

Epithelioid mesothelioma cells are usually larger than normal mesothelial cells, having large nuclei with various nuclear anomalies and prominent nucleoli. Neoplastic mesothelial cells may appear to be non-cohesive (Fig. 2.29) and are gathered in spherical (Fig. 2.30), papillary (Fig. 2.31), or pseudoglandular patterns (Fig. 2.32). Sometimes, neoplastic mesothelial cells can assume a rhabdoid appearance (Fig. 2.33), or they may show clear-cell (Fig. 2.34) or deciduous features (Fig. 2.35). In some cases neoplastic mesothelial cells show marked cytoplasmic vacuolization (Fig. 2.36).

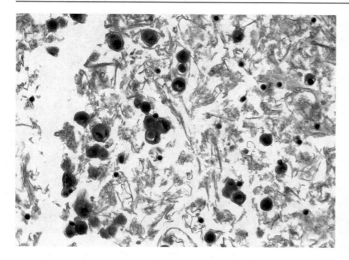

Fig. 2.29 Single mesothelioma cells. H&E (high magnification)

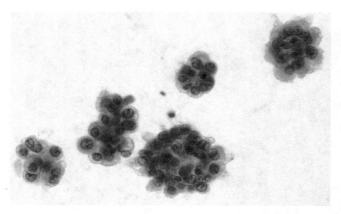

Fig. 2.30 Mesothelioma spherical structures. H&E (high magnification)

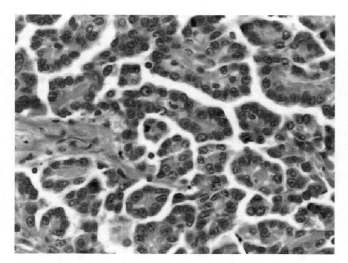

Fig. 2.31 Papillary mesothelioma. H&E (high magnification)

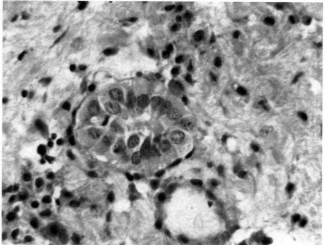

Fig. 2.32 Pseudoglandular mesothelioma. H&E (high magnification)

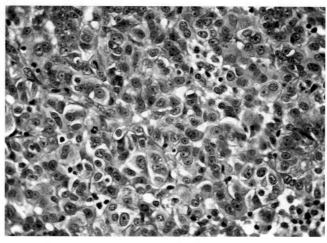

Fig. 2.33 Rhabdoid mesothelioma. H&E (high magnification)

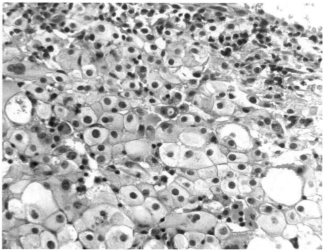

Fig. 2.34 Clear-cell mesothelioma. H&E (high magnification)

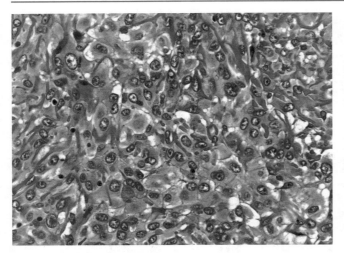

Fig. 2.35   Deciduoid mesothelioma. H&E (high magnification)

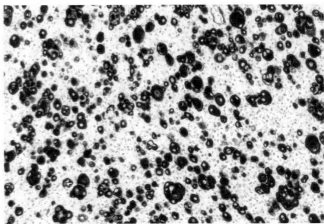

Fig. 2.37   Mesothelioma. CK5 immunostain (high magnification)

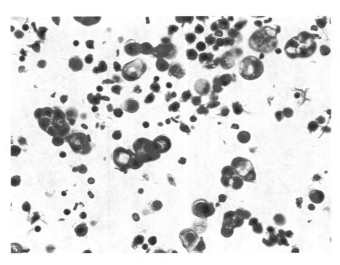

Fig. 2.36   Signet-ring cell mesothelioma. H&E (high magnification)

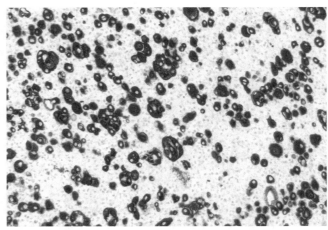

Fig. 2.38   Mesothelioma. CK7 immunostain (high magnification)

We must emphasize that epithelioid mesothelioma and all of its cytomorphologic variants have the same immunophenotype. Neoplastic mesothelial cells express vimentin and several cytokeratin markers, such as CK5 (Fig. 2.37), CK6, CK7 (Fig. 2.38), CK8, CK18, and CK 19, whereas other cytokeratins (CK4, CK14, and CK17) can be variably expressed. Moreover, mesothelioma cells are positive for calretinin (Fig. 2.39), podoplanin (Fig. 2.40), WT-1 (Fig. 2.41), and caveolin-1. Membrane with mild cytoplasmic positivity with EMA (Fig. 2.42), HMFGP, HBME-1 (Fig. 2.43), and mesothelin (Fig. 2.44) is also characteristic of epithelioid mesothelioma. The neoplastic cells are also immunoreactive with antibodies to thrombomodulin, cadherin N, CD44H, AMAD-2, and GLUT-1 (Fig. 2.45). These markers may also be positive in some types of carcinoma.

Negative cell-immunostaining reactions can be observed with desmin (Fig. 2.46) and BAP-1. Also, IMP-3 is usually

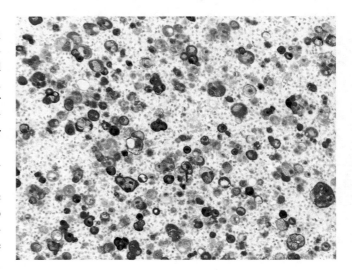

Fig. 2.39   Mesothelioma. Calretinin immunostain (high magnification)

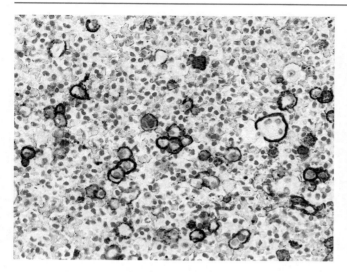

Fig. 2.40 Mesothelioma. Podoplanin immunostain (high magnification)

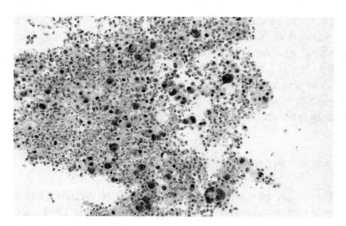

Fig. 2.41 Mesothelioma. WT-1 immunostain (high magnification)

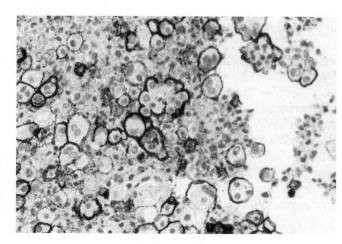

Fig. 2.42 Mesothelioma. EMA immunostain (high magnification)

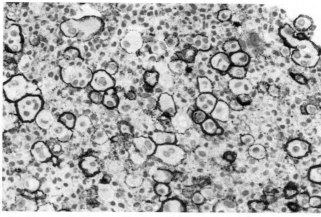

Fig. 2.43 Mesothelioma. HBME-1 immunostain (high magnification)

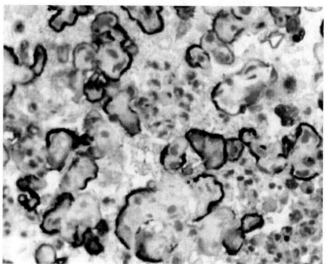

Fig. 2.44 Mesothelioma. Mesothelin immunostain (high magnification)

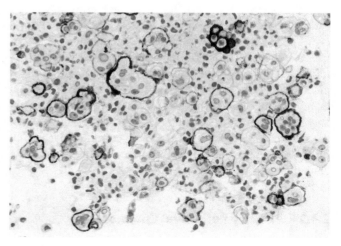

Fig. 2.45 Mesothelioma. GLUT-1 immunostain (high magnification)

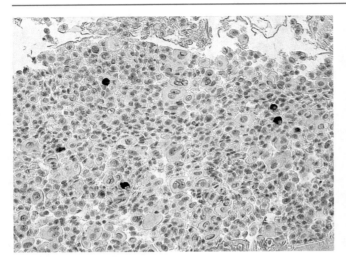

Fig. 2.46 Mesothelioma. Desmin immunostain (high magnification)

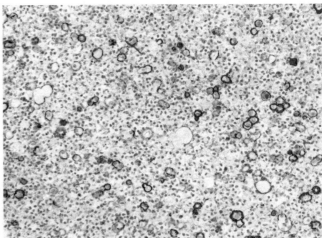

Fig. 2.48 Mesothelioma. CEA immunostain (high magnification)

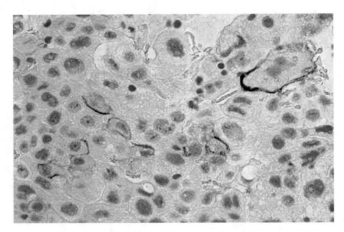

Fig. 2.47 Mesothelioma. CA15.3 immunostain (high magnification)

negative in neoplastic mesothelial cells. No carcinoma-associated markers, such as ESA, ERA, TAG B72.3, claudin, etc., are expressed in mesothelioma. Antibodies directed to carbohydrate antigens, such as CA15.3 (Fig. 2.47), CA19.9, or CA125, can stain the membranes of epithelioid mesothelial cells in about 15–20% of mesothelioma cases. The CEA immunostaining is considered negative, even if rare epithelioid mesothelioma cells with positivity limited to the cell membrane are found (Fig. 2.48). This phenomenon is probably due to interactions (or perhaps a cross-reaction) between the antibody and the high content of glycosaminoglycan and/or hyaluronic acid in the cytoplasmic membranes of some epithelioid mesothelioma cells.

2.4.2 Primary Peritoneal Carcinoma

The cytologic diagnosis of this neoplasia is very difficult because of the close relationship between serous carcinomas and mesotheliomas in terms of the growth pattern, cytomorphology, and immunophenotype. This neoplasia shows a growth pattern similar to that of mesothelioma, but has an immunophenotype similar to that of serous tumors of the ovary, i.e., positivity for CK7, WT-1, PAX-8, CA125, and EMA. Furthermore, some neoplastic cells can express estrogen receptors. Therefore, the diagnosis of primary peritoneal carcinoma must be made only in the absence of an ovarian primary.

2.4.3 Primary Pleural Lymphoma

Pleural lymphomas are rare, comprising two different specific entities, namely, primary effusion lymphoma (PEL) and diffuse large B-cell lymphoma associated with chronic inflammation (DLBCL-CI). However, a number of distinct forms of hematologic malignancies may involve the pleura, usually as secondary involvement from a nodal, extranodal, or bone marrow-based disease.

Primary effusion lymphoma (PEL) This is a neoplasm of large B cells, which occurs in the serous effusion fluid, without detectable lymph node tumor masses. PEL usually is a lymphoma associated with the herpes virus of Kaposi's sarcoma (HHV-8) and occurs particularly in cases of acquired immunodeficiency disease. However, PEL has been documented in HIV-negative allograft recipients. Primary effusion lymphoma predominantly involves the pleura, although it can also involve the peritoneum or pericardium, or it may be present as multicavitary disease.

Cytologically, tumor cells in the effusion can appear as discohesive large malignant lymphoid cells with immunoblastic features, including large vesicular nuclei and prominent nucleoli, which are present along with plasmablastic

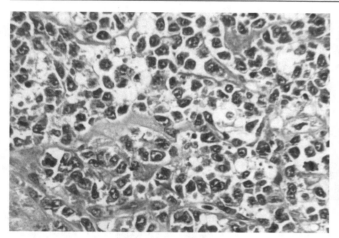

Fig. 2.49 Plasmablastic cells in PEL H&E (high magnification)

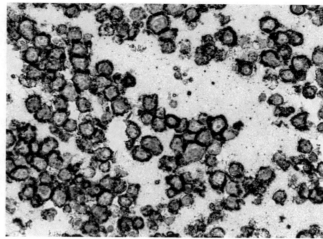

Fig. 2.51 PEL CD45 immunostain (high magnification)

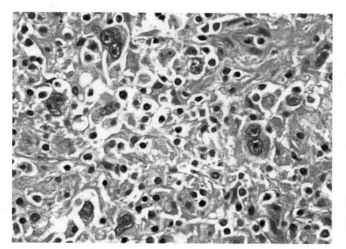

Fig. 2.50 Reed–Sternberg-like cells in PEL H&E (high magnification)

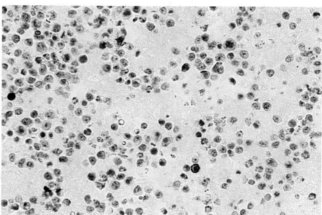

Fig. 2.52 PEL CD20 immunostain (high magnification)

elements (Fig. 2.49). Multinucleated cells, sometimes with a Reed–Sternberg cell appearance (Fig. 2.50), may be seen in some cases.

Neoplastic cells express CD45 (Fig. 2.51), whereas markers of the B-cell lineage, such as CD19, CD20 (Fig. 2.52), and CD79a, and those of the T-cell population are usually negative. Surface immunoglobulins are not expressed, whereas cytoplasmic immunoglobulins are occasionally present in some cells (Fig. 2.53). This distinct immunophenotype is due to a defect in transcriptional activation, as demonstrated by immunohistochemical negativity for PU.1, Oct 2, and BOB.1. CD10 and bcl-6 are also absent, whereas CD30, CD38, CD138 (Fig. 2.54), MUM1/IRF4 (Fig. 2.55), and the antigens associated with HHV-8 (Fig. 2.56) are expressed. In some cases, the EBV marking is present (exclusivity only for EBNA-1 and negativity for EBNA-2, LMP-1, and LMP-2). Very rare cases with cytoplasmic expression of CD3, CD7, and CD56 have also been described.

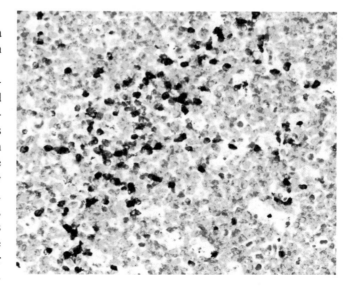

Fig. 2.53 PEL cytoplasmic kappa light-chain immunostain (high magnification)

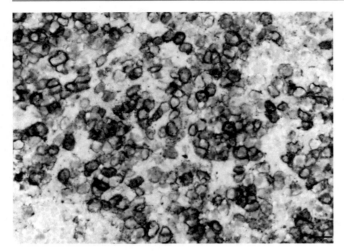

Fig. 2.54 PEL CD138 immunostain (high magnification)

Diffuse large B-cell lymphoma associated with chronic inflammation This lymphoma morphologically shows immunoblastic features (Fig. 2.57), and it is positive for CD45, CD19, CD20 (Fig. 2.58), CD79a, PAX-5, and, in many cases, CD30 (Fig. 2.59) and MUM1/IRF4 (Fig. 2.60). Markers of germinal center cells, CD10 and bcl-6 (Fig. 2.61), are usually negative. The characteristics of EBV infection are highlighted in the neoplastic elements, because these cells show an intense positivity for EBER (Fig. 2.62), EBNA-2, and, sometimes, for LMP-1.

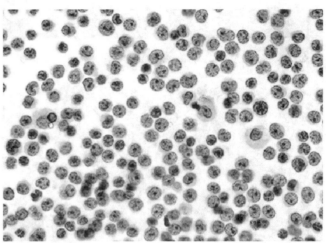

Fig. 2.57 Lymphoma associated with chronic inflammation. H&E (high magnification)

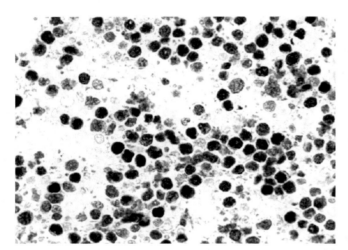

Fig. 2.55 PEL MUM1/IRF4 immunostain (high magnification)

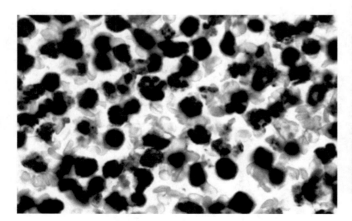

Fig. 2.56 PEL HHV8 immunostain (high magnification)

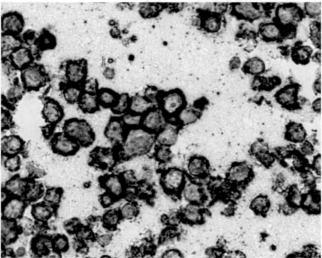

Fig. 2.58 Lymphoma associated with chronic inflammation. CD20 immunostain (high magnification)

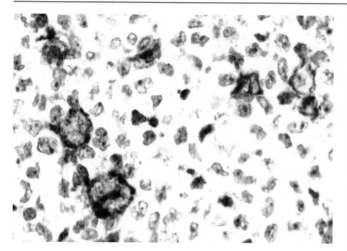

Fig. 2.59 Lymphoma associated with chronic inflammation. CD30 immunostain (high magnification)

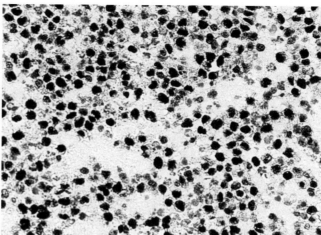

Fig. 2.62 Lymphoma associated with chronic inflammation. EBER (high magnification)

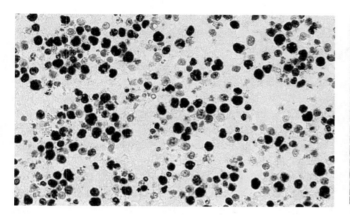

Fig. 2.60 Lymphoma associated with chronic inflammation. MUM1/IRF4 immunostain (high magnification)

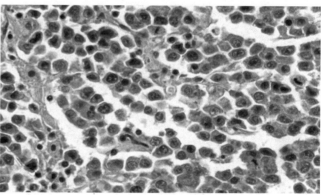

Fig. 2.63 Plasmacytoid/plasmoblastic differentiation. H&E (high magnification)

Some cases show plasmacytoid/plasmoblastic cell differentiation (Fig. 2.63), and, therefore, cells are negative for CD20 (Fig. 2.64) and CD79 markers, whereas they express CD138 (Fig. 2.65) and cytoplasmic immunoglobulins with clonal restriction. EBV-infected cells can be identified by their EBER positivity (Fig. 2.66). Epstein–Barr virus can also promote the expression of T-cell line markers (CD2, CD3, CD4, and CD7) in transformed cells.

2.5 Metastatic Serous Effusions

Serous cavities are frequent sites of metastasis; therefore, serous effusions may contain neoplastic cells that originated in other sites.

Metastatic serous effusion shows a difference in frequency, depending on the primary site and gender. Also, the

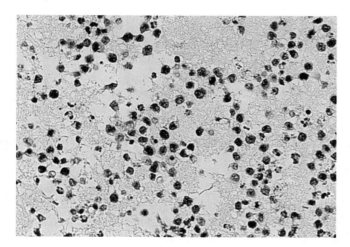

Fig. 2.61 Lymphoma associated with chronic inflammation. Bcl-6 immunostain (high magnification)

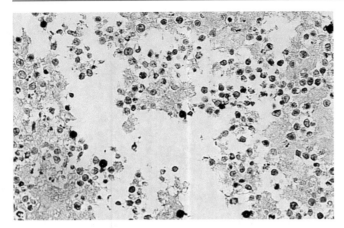

Fig. 2.64 Plasmacytoid/plasmoblastic differentiation. CD20 immunostain (high magnification)

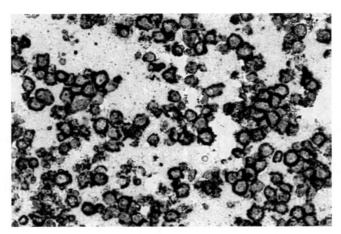

Fig. 2.65 Plasmacytoid/plasmoblastic differentiation. CD138 immunostain (high magnification)

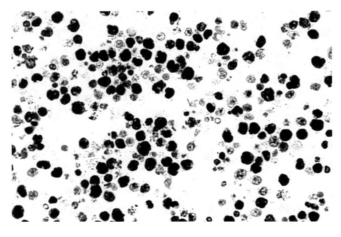

Fig. 2.66 Plasmacytoid/plasmoblastic differentiation. EBER (high magnification)

distribution of metastatic involvement has differences in frequency depending on their localization (pleural, pericardial, or peritoneal).

In men, metastatic pleural effusions are most commonly caused by lung cancer; the adenocarcinoma variant of lung cancer is the most frequent due to its common peripheral localization in the lung. Neoplastic cells of the digestive system, lymphomas/leukemias, and melanoma are next in the frequency of metastatic pleural effusions. In women, the most frequent source of a malignant pleural effusion is carcinoma of the breast, followed by the lung, ovary, and gastrointestinal tract.

As to metastatic peritoneal effusions, the most frequent tumors in men are those from the gastrointestinal tract, followed by those of pulmonary, pancreatic, and hepatic origin. Secondary peritoneal effusions in women have a more common origin in the ovary, followed by the digestive system, uterus, breast, pancreas, liver, and biliary tract.

Secondary pericardial effusion in men is most commonly caused by lung adenocarcinoma, whereas in women it is breast cancer.

Carcinomas arising from certain anatomic sites may exhibit some specific cytologic characteristics in serous effusions, despite the presence of considerable overlapping features. Thus, in secondary malignant effusions, the cell size, degree of cohesiveness, form of aggregation, and cell distribution, among other features, may suggest a specific diagnosis and site of origin.

In the case of about 20% of neoplastic serous effusions, the primary cancer is unknown or occult at the time of initial investigation. The diagnosis is usually facilitated when the primary tumor is known, whereas, in the case of an unknown primary origin, the diagnosis requires a rigorous clinicopathologic correlation and the use of various ancillary techniques.

2.5.1 Lung Adenocarcinoma Cells in Serous Effusion

Exfoliated cells from lung adenocarcinoma can be single and non-cohesive (Fig. 2.67) or clustered in irregular spherical (Fig. 2.68), papillary (Fig. 2.69), or glandular structures (Fig. 2.70). The neoplastic cells can show cytoplasmic vacuoles, prominent nucleoli, and multinucleation.

Lung adenocarcinoma cells express CK7 (Fig. 2.71), TTF1 (Fig. 2.72), napsin A (Fig. 2.73), and most epithelium-related cancer antigens, such as CEA (Fig. 2.74), ESA (Fig. 2.75), and ERA. Neoplastic cells with vacuolated cytoplasm usually are stained by anti-surfactant antibody (Fig. 2.76), suggesting their pneumocyte type II origin. Obviously, mesothelial cell marker immunostains are negative.

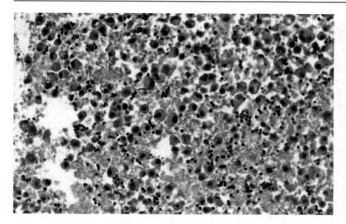

Fig. 2.67 Single non-cohesive lung adenocarcinoma cells. H&E (high magnification)

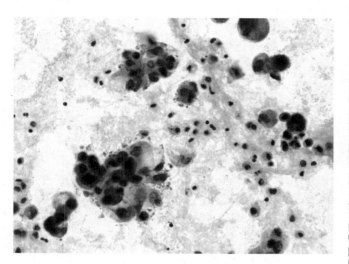

Fig. 2.68 Spherical aggregate of lung adenocarcinoma cells. H&E (high magnification)

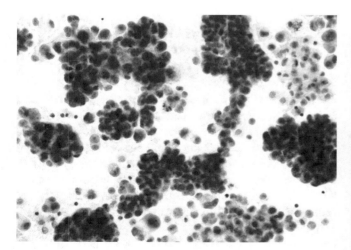

Fig. 2.69 Papillary aggregate of lung adenocarcinoma cells. H&E (high magnification)

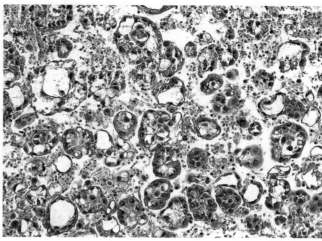

Fig. 2.70 Acinic structure of lung adenocarcinoma cells. H&E (high magnification)

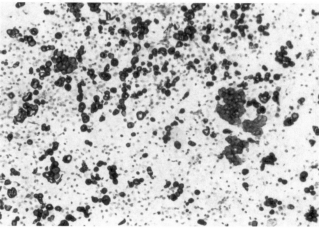

Fig. 2.71 Lung adenocarcinoma cells. CK7 immunostain (high magnification)

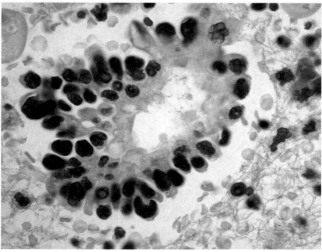

Fig. 2.72 Lung adenocarcinoma cells. TTF-1 immunostain (high magnification)

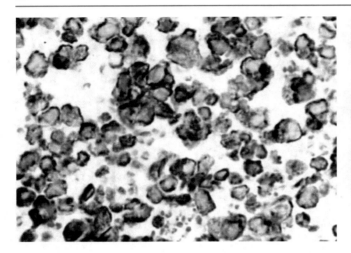

Fig. 2.73 Lung adenocarcinoma cells. Napsin A immunostain (high magnification)

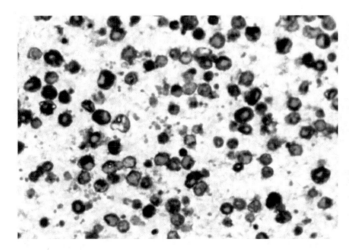

Fig. 2.74 Lung adenocarcinoma cells. CEA immunostain (high magnification)

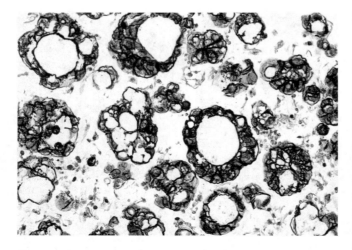

Fig. 2.75 Lung adenocarcinoma cells. ESA immunostain (high magnification)

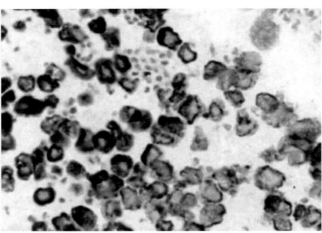

Fig. 2.76 Lung metastatic adenocarcinoma. Surfactant immunostain (high magnification)

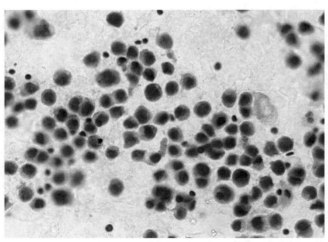

Fig. 2.77 Lung squamous neoplastic cells. H&E (high magnification)

2.5.2 Lung Squamous Carcinoma Cells in Serous Effusion

Squamous carcinoma can involve serous tissue, but the presence of exfoliated cells in serous effusions is an uncommon event. Squamous neoplastic cells are seen singly (Fig. 2.77), in small sheets or in large syncytial clusters. Well-differentiated or keratinizing carcinoma cells do not require immunocytochemistry for the diagnosis, whereas poorly differentiated tumor cells usually are indistinguishable from those of adenocarcinoma and mesothelioma. Nonkeratinized cells are usually round, and they may form cohesive clusters. Sometimes, cytoplasmic vacuoles may be seen. Positive immunostains for CK5 (Fig. 2.78) or CK5/6, p40 (Fig. 2.79), p63, and desmocollin-3 (Fig. 2.80) help to make the diagnosis. Neoplastic cells are negative with mesothelioma markers, TTF-1, or napsin A. Cells are positive for CK7 in rare cases.

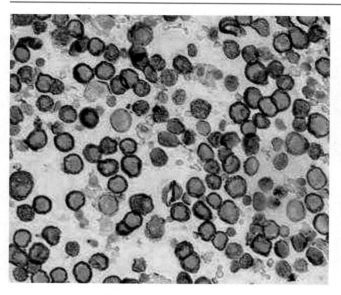

Fig. 2.78 Lung squamous neoplastic cells. CK5 immunostain (high magnification)

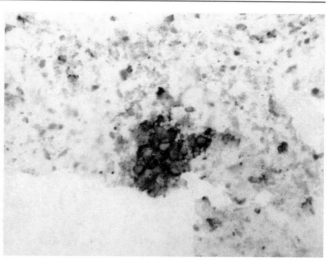

Fig. 2.80 Lung squamous neoplastic cells. Desmocollin-3 immunostain (high magnification)

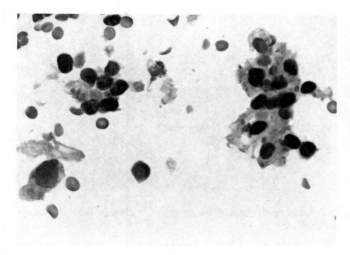

Fig. 2.79 Lung squamous neoplastic cells. p40 immunostain (high magnification)

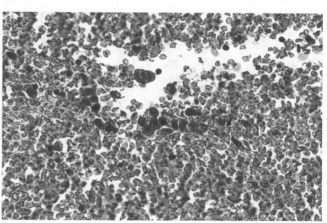

Fig. 2.81 Lung neuroendocrine carcinoma. H&E (high magnification)

2.5.3 Lung Neuroendocrine Carcinoma Cells in Serous Effusion

Neuroendocrine neoplastic cells usually are small and cuboidal, with scant cytoplasm and round nuclei without nucleoli. Chromatin can show a "salt-and-pepper" appearance or exhibit Azzopardi's phenomenon. The neoplastic cells can be single, arranged in "Indian file" (Fig. 2.81), or in small clusters. Sometimes, neuroendocrine neoplastic cells are large with conspicuous nucleoli. Small and large neuroendocrine cells show positivity for chromogranin A (Fig. 2.82), synaptophysin, CD56, TTF-1 (Fig. 2.83), and neuron-specific enolase. Neoplastic cells express low-molecular-

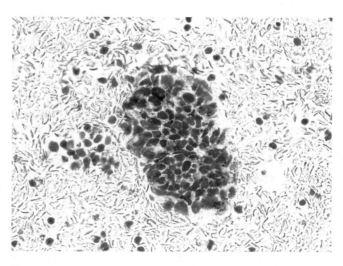

Fig. 2.82 Lung neuroendocrine carcinoma. Chromogranin A immunostain (high magnification)

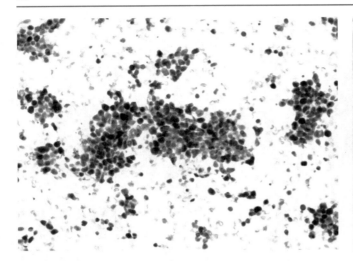

Fig. 2.83 Lung neuroendocrine carcinoma. TTF-1 immunostain (high magnification)

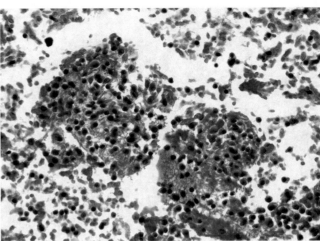

Fig. 2.85 Morulae of ductal breast carcinoma. H&E (high magnification)

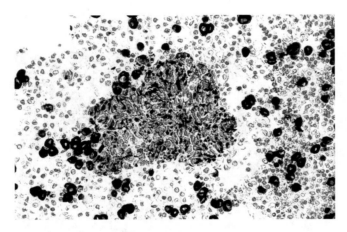

Fig. 2.84 Lung neuroendocrine carcinoma. CK8 immunostain (high magnification)

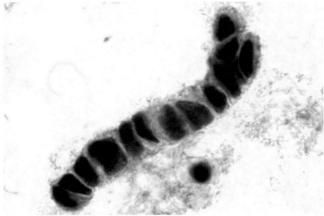

Fig. 2.86 Small chain of lobular breast carcinoma. H&E (high magnification)

weight cytokeratins CK8 (Fig. 2.84), CK18, and CK19 with a typical dot-like cytoplasmic stain.

2.5.4 Breast Cancer Cells in Serous Effusion

Neoplastic cells from ductal carcinoma are present as large clusters, numerous spherical aggregates ("cannon balls"), or papillae or sometimes singly. They usually have a monomorphic aspect with non-vacuolated abundant cytoplasm, irregular nuclei, and multiple nucleoli (Fig. 2.85).

Neoplastic cells from lobular breast cancer usually are single or arranged in small chains. Morphologically, they show scant cytoplasm with small vacuoles compressing hyperchromatic nuclei (Fig. 2.86).

The immunocytochemistry is similar in ductal and lobular breast carcinoma: positivity for CK7 (Fig. 2.87) and GATA-3 (Fig. 2.88). Most neoplastic cells express

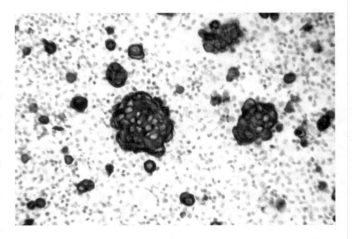

Fig. 2.87 Ductal breast carcinoma. CK7 immunostain (high magnification)

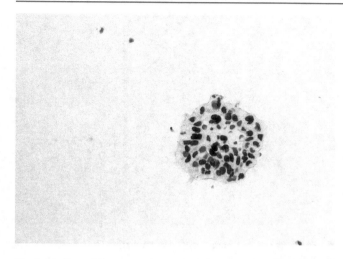

Fig. 2.88 Ductal breast carcinoma. GATA-3 immunostain (high magnification)

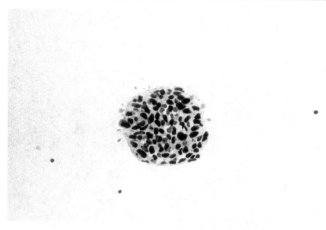

Fig. 2.90 Ductal breast carcinoma. Estrogen receptors immunostain (high magnification)

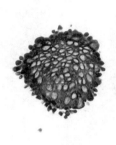

Fig. 2.89 Ductal breast carcinoma. Mammaglobin immunostain (high magnification)

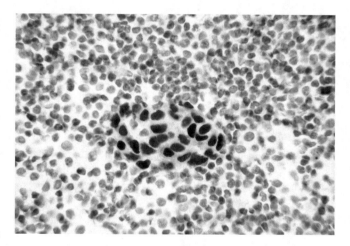

Fig. 2.91 Ductal breast carcinoma. Progesterone receptors immunostain (high magnification)

mammaglobin (Fig. 2.89) and gross cystic disease fluid proteins (GCDFP-15), whereas CK20, p63, and mesothelial markers are negative. Cytologic samples can be used for assessing the presence of estrogen (Fig. 2.90) and progesterone receptors (Fig. 2.91) and HER-2 protein (Fig. 2.92).

2.5.5 Gastric Adenocarcinoma Cells in Serous Effusion

Here the neoplastic cells usually have scant cytoplasm, or they sometimes show cytoplasmic vacuoles imparting a signet-ring appearance to the cells (Fig. 2.93). The serous effusion is usually highly cellular, with small-cell clusters and numerous isolated adenocarcinoma cells. Neoplastic cells express CK7 (Fig. 2.94) and/or CK20 (Fig. 2.95), or only LMW-CK (CK8, CK18, CK19). HepPar antigen

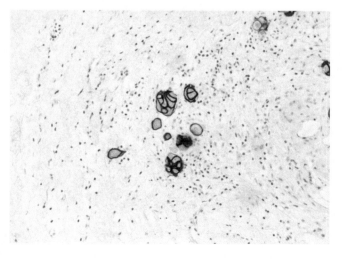

Fig. 2.92 Ductal breast carcinoma. HER-2 protein immunostain (high magnification)

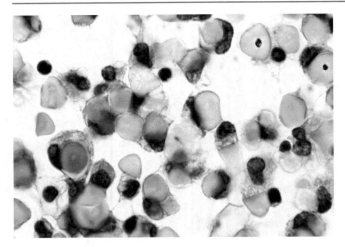

Fig. 2.93 Gastric carcinoma cells. H&E (high magnification)

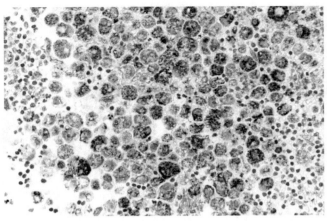

Fig. 2.96 Gastric carcinoma cells. HepPar antigen immunostain (high magnification)

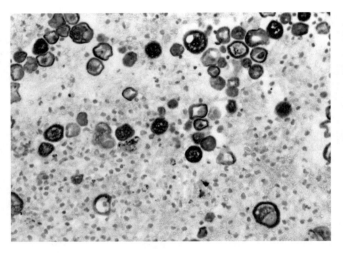

Fig. 2.94 Gastric carcinoma cells. CK7 immunostain (high magnification)

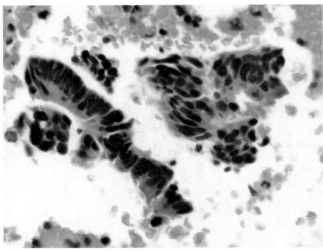

Fig. 2.97 Large bowel carcinoma. H&E (high magnification)

(Fig. 2.96), pS2 protein, and carbohydrate antigen markers can be present in gastric cancer cells.

2.5.6 Large Bowel Adenocarcinoma Cells in Serous Effusion

These neoplastic cells usually form glandular, acinar, or papillary structures. The cells are large and columnar with nuclear palisades (Fig. 2.97) and intracytoplasmic vacuoles containing mucin. Pleomorphic signet-ring cells can be present.

Usually, large bowel adenocarcinoma cells are positive for CK20 (Fig. 2.98), CDX-2 (Fig. 2.99), CEA, and villin. Some neoplastic cells can express CK7 (Fig. 2.100) and carbohydrate antigens (CA125, CA15.3, CA19.9, B72.3).

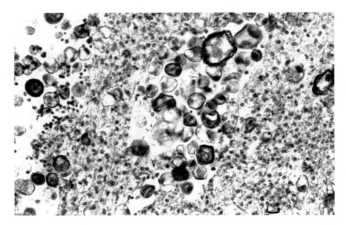

Fig. 2.95 Gastric carcinoma cells. CK20 immunostain (high magnification)

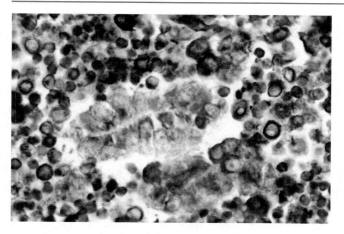

Fig. 2.98 Large bowel carcinoma. CK20 immunostain (high magnification)

2.5.7 Normal and Neoplastic Endometrial Cells in Serous Effusion

Morules and aggregates of normal endometrial cells can be observed in serous effusion, which usually is ascites caused by endometriosis. Endometrioid carcinoma cells are present as single and clustered small cuboidal neoplastic cells with scant cytoplasm, enlarged monomorphic or pleomorphic nuclei, coarse chromatin, and prominent nucleoli (Fig. 2.101). The neoplastic cells express vimentin, CK7 (Fig. 2.102), CK8, CK18, CK19, ESA (Ber-Ep4), EMA, and TAG B72.3. Focal positive cells for CK5, CK6, CK14, CK17, and PAX-8 (Fig. 2.103) can be seen. Estrogen receptor (ER), PgR, and β-catenin can be positive, whereas p53, CEA, and PTEN are negative in well- and moderately differentiated adenocarcinomas. Cytologic preparations can be used for assessment of the instability of the microsatellites MLH, PMS2, MSH2, and MSH6.

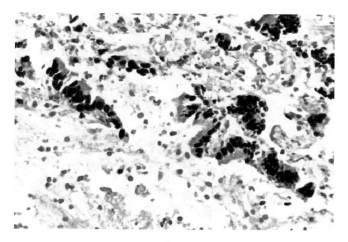

Fig. 2.99 Large bowel carcinoma. CDX-2 immunostain (high magnification)

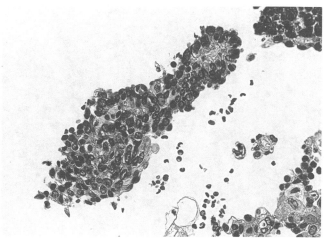

Fig. 2.101 Endometrioid endometrial carcinoma. H&E (high magnification)

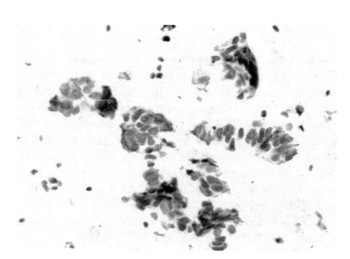

Fig. 2.100 Large bowel carcinoma. CK7 immunostain (high magnification)

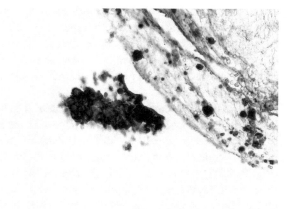

Fig. 2.102 Endometrioid endometrial carcinoma. CK7 immunostain (high magnification)

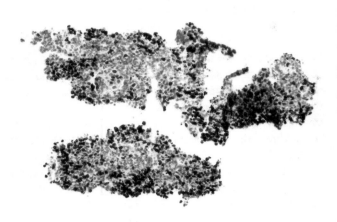

Fig. 2.103 Endometrioid endometrial carcinoma. PAX-8 immunostain (high magnification)

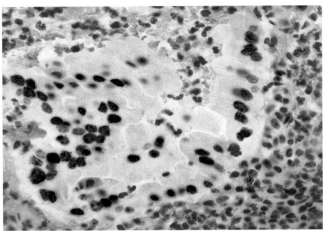

Fig. 2.105 Serous papillary endometrial carcinoma. p53 immunostain (high magnification)

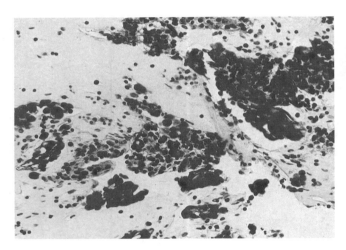

Fig. 2.104 Serous papillary endometrial carcinoma. H&E (high magnification)

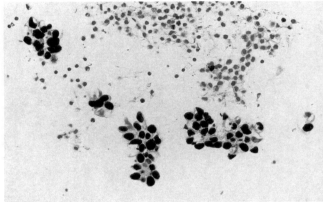

Fig. 2.106 Serous papillary endometrial carcinoma. PTEN immunostain (high magnification)

Clustered small cuboidal cells with scant cytoplasm and enlarged hyperchromatic nuclei with inconspicuous nucleoli characterize serous papillary endometrial carcinoma (Fig. 2.104), whereas clear-cell endometrial carcinoma shows single and clustered pleomorphic malignant cells with clear cytoplasm.

Serous papillary and clear-cell endometrial carcinomas exhibit features that are similar to those seen in the endometrioid type. However, cells are different from those of endometrioid cancer by having intense positivity for p53 (Fig. 2.105), PTEN (Fig. 2.106), β-catenin, MLH1, MSH2, MSH6, and PMS2. Serous papillary carcinoma shows CEA-positive cells, whereas clear-cell carcinoma is positive for HNF-1β (hepatocyte nuclear factor-1β).

2.5.8   Neoplastic Cervical Cells in Serous Effusion

Uterine cervix adenocarcinoma cells as well as those of non-keratinizing squamous cell carcinoma (Fig. 2.107) are seen in sheet-like arrangements (Fig. 2.108), whereas cells derived from keratinizing squamous cell carcinoma are often present singly or in syncytial aggregates. Cells from adenocarcinoma usually have abundant thin cytoplasm, eccentrically located nuclei, slight to moderate hyperchromasia with irregularly distributed chromatin, and large nucleoli. Immunocytochemistry is positive for CK7, CK8, CK18, CK19, CEA (Fig. 2.109), p16, EMA, and MUC5AC. Some neoplastic cells express CK4, CK6, CK14, and CK17. The intestinal variant of adenocarcinoma is CDX-2 positive, but CK20-negative.

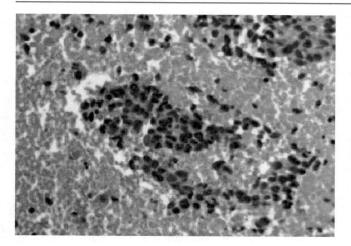

Fig. 2.107 Cervix adenocarcinoma. H&E (high magnification)

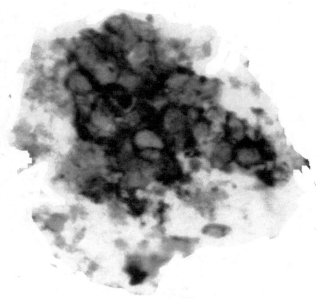

Fig. 2.110 Squamous cell carcinoma. CK5 immunostain (high magnification)

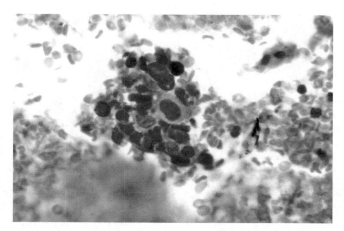

Fig. 2.108 Nonkeratinizing squamous cell carcinoma. H&E (high magnification)

Nonkeratinizing squamous carcinoma cells have a moderate amount of cytoplasm, hyperchromatic round to oval or irregularly shaped nuclei, coarsely granular and irregular chromatin, and conspicuous nucleoli. Keratinizing squamous carcinoma cells have round/oval/bizarre shapes, with dense eosinophilic cytoplasm, and round/oval nuclei with considerable variations in form and size. Neoplastic squamous cells express CK4, CK5 (Fig. 2.110), CK6, CK8, CK13, CK14, CK16, CK19, CEA, and p16. Some cells or small clusters can be positive for CK7, CK10, CK11, and CK17.

2.5.9 Ovarian Serous Carcinoma Cells in Serous Effusion

Neoplastic cells can have different sizes with small vacuoles that may be due to the presence of glycogen. Most neoplastic cells have a cytomorphologic mesothelial-like aspect. Typical acinar or papillary cohesive clusters and isolated cells can be observed (Fig. 2.111).

Immunocytochemistry shows positivity for CK7 (Fig. 2.112), WT-1 (Fig. 2.113), PAX-8 (Fig. 2.114), and CA125. Some neoplastic cells can express CK5 (Fig. 2.115), CA15.3, and CA19.9. A characteristic is the immunoreaction for B72.3 (Fig. 2.116) that stains only the cytoplasmic membrane and EMA, which stains the cytoplasm. Investigations for the presence of hormonal receptor, ERα, ERβ, and PgR are usually carried out for tailored therapy.

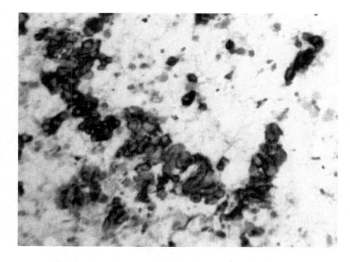

Fig. 2.109 Squamous cell carcinoma. CEA immunostain (high magnification)

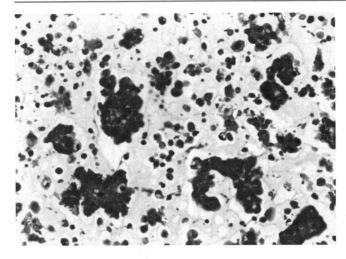

Fig. 2.111   Ovary serous carcinoma. H&E (high magnification)

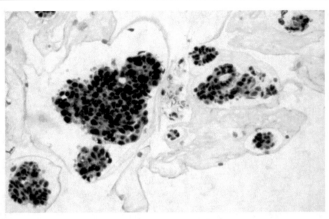

Fig. 2.114   Ovary serous carcinoma. PAX-8 immunostain (high magnification)

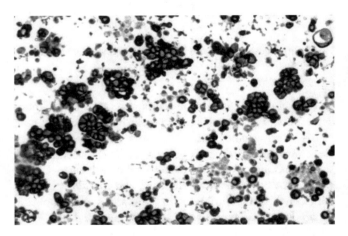

Fig. 2.112   Ovary serous carcinoma. CK7 immunostain (high magnification)

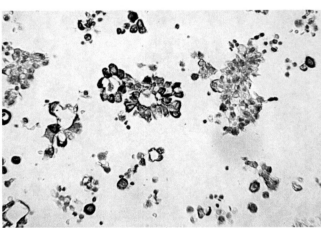

Fig. 2.115   Ovary serous carcinoma. CK5 immunostain (high magnification)

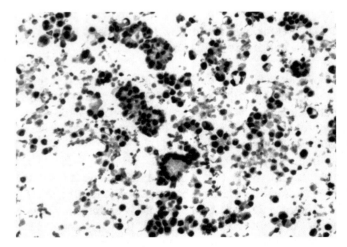

Fig. 2.113   Ovary serous carcinoma. WT-1 immunostain (high magnification)

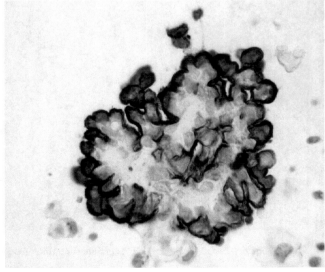

Fig. 2.116   Ovary serous carcinoma. B72.3 immunostain (high magnification)

2.5.10 Ovarian Mucinous Carcinoma Cells in Serous Effusion

Neoplastic cells show a vacuolated cytoplasm containing mucin and, usually, eccentric nuclei (Fig. 2.117). Smears usually are cellular and show single and clustered tumor cells that are positive for CK7 (Fig. 2.118), B72.3, HAM56, cytoplasmic EMA (Fig. 2.119), and EpCam. Neoplastic cells express CK20, WT-1, PAX-8, CDX-2 (Fig. 2.120), CEA, MUC-2, and MUC-5AC in different proportions.

2.5.11 Germ-Cell Tumor Cells in Serous Effusion

Neoplastic cells from germ-cell tumors can be present in serous effusions. Cells from endodermal sinus (yolk sac) tumor (Fig. 2.121), embryonal carcinoma (Fig. 2.122), and choriocar-

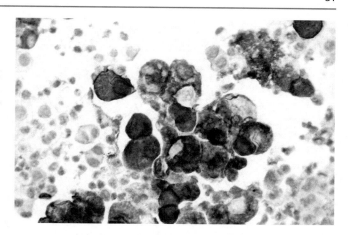

Fig. 2.119 Ovary mucinous carcinoma. EMA immunostain (high magnification)

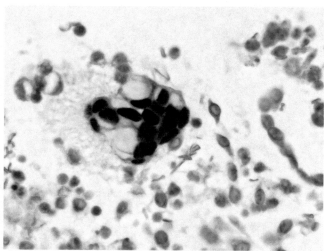

Fig. 2.120 Ovary mucinous carcinoma. CDX-2 immunostain (high magnification)

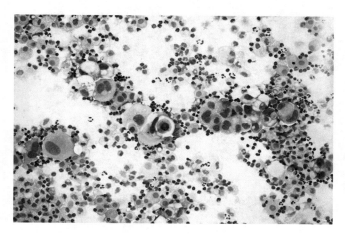

Fig. 2.117 Ovary mucinous carcinoma. Papanicolaou stain (high magnification)

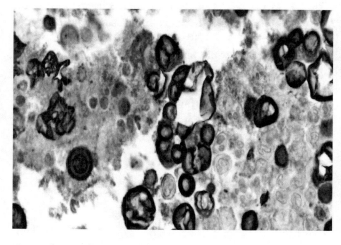

Fig. 2.118 Ovary mucinous carcinoma. CK7 immunostain (high magnification)

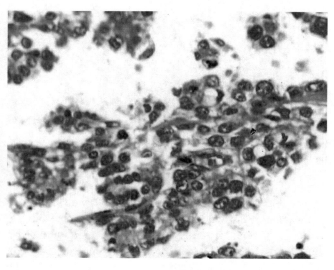

Fig. 2.121 Yolk sac tumor. H&E (high magnification)

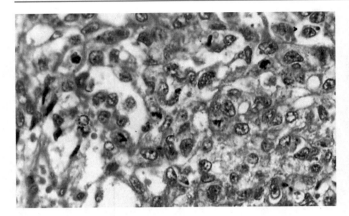

Fig. 2.122   Embryonal carcinoma. H&E (high magnification)

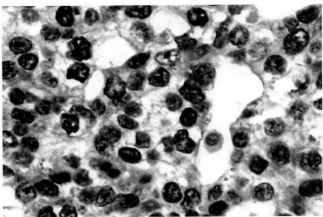

Fig. 2.125   Yolk sac tumor. SALL-4 immunostain (high magnification)

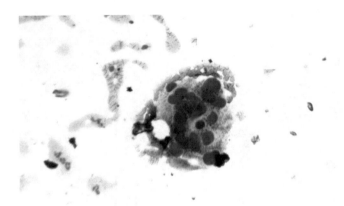

Fig. 2.123   Choriocarcinoma. H&E (high magnification)

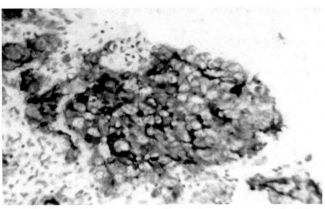

Fig. 2.126   Embryonal carcinoma. PLAP immunostain (high magnification)

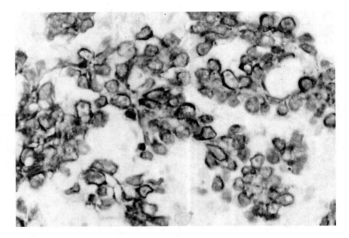

Fig. 2.124   Yolk sac tumor. Glypican-3 immunostain (high magnification)

min, β1-PS, and ferritin. Cells of embryonal carcinoma express SALL-4, OCT4, PLAP (Fig. 2.126), CD30 (Fig. 2.127), CK7, CK8, and CK18. Rare cells are positive for hPL and α-fetoprotein. Choriocarcinoma shows positivity for PLAP, SALL-4 (Fig. 2.128), CK8, CK18, and CK19.

Seminoma/dysgerminoma cells are non-cohesive and uniform, and they resemble large mesothelial cells with large nucleoli. Neoplastic cells usually express dot-like PLAP, OCT-4, SALL-4, podoplanin (Fig. 2.129), CD117 (Fig. 2.130), NANOG, SOX-17, CD143, and VASA. Occasionally, cells are stained with CK8 and/or CK18 (in a dot-like pattern).

2.5.12 Hepatocellular Carcinoma Cells in Serous Effusion

Hepatocellular carcinoma cells are polygonal and have abundant granular cytoplasm and large round/oval nuclei with prominent nucleoli or macronucleoli. In serous effusions, they are single or form large irregular clusters (Fig. 2.131)

cinoma (Fig. 2.123) are large pleomorphic cells with pale, finely granular chromatin and prominent, often multiple nucleoli.

Yolk sac tumor cells are positive for glypican-3 (Fig. 2.124), SALL-4 (Fig. 2.125), and low-molecular-weight cytokeratins. Different numbers of neoplastic cells can be immunostained by PLAP, α-fetoprotein, α-1-antitripsin, albu-

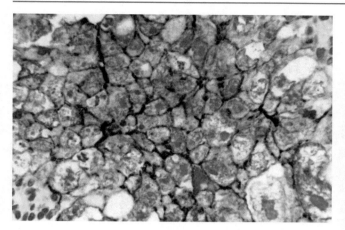

Fig. 2.127 Embryonal carcinoma. CD30 immunostain (high magnification)

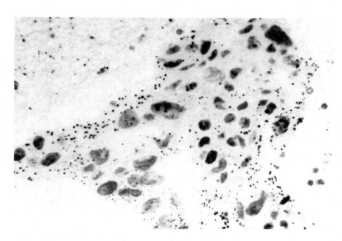

Fig. 2.128 Embryonal carcinoma. SALL-4 immunostain (high magnification)

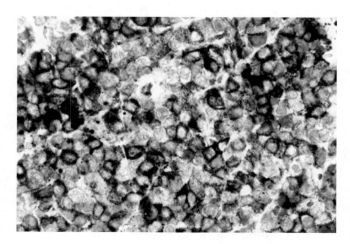

Fig. 2.129 Dysgerminoma. Podoplanin immunostain (high magnification)

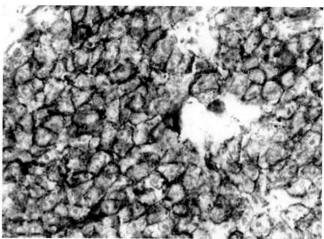

Fig. 2.130 Dysgerminoma. CD117 immunostain (high magnification)

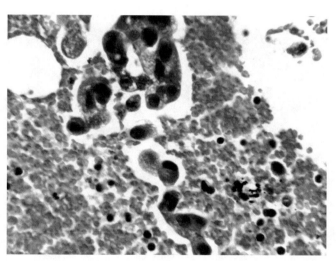

Fig. 2.131 Hepatocellular carcinoma. H&E (high magnification)

and show positive immunostaining for CK8 (Fig. 2.132), CK18, HepPar-1, Glypican-3 (Fig. 2.133), cytoplasmic TTF-1 (Fig. 2.134), and α-fetoprotein, whereas CK20 is negative and CK7 is expressed only in the lamellar variant.

2.5.13 Urothelial Carcinoma Cells in Serous Effusion

High-grade urothelial carcinoma cells can be observed in serous effusions as single or cohesive irregular clusters (Fig. 2.135). Neoplastic cells usually have a granular cytoplasm, oval nuclei, and prominent nucleoli. Their cellular urothelial origin can be determined by the expression of CK7

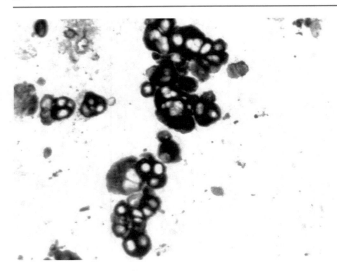

Fig. 2.132 Hepatocellular carcinoma. CK8 immunostain (high magnification)

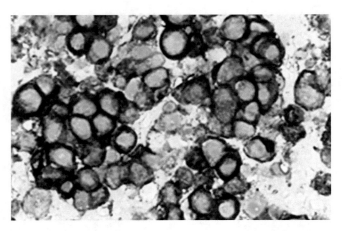

Fig. 2.133 Hepatocellular carcinoma. Glypican-3 immunostain (high magnification)

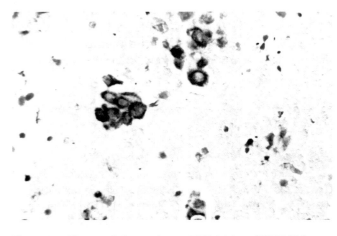

Fig. 2.134 Hepatocellular carcinoma. TTF-1 (clone 8G7G3/1) immunostain (high magnification)

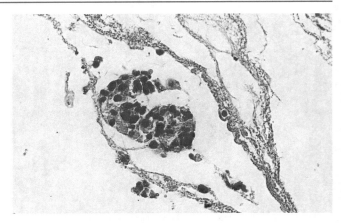

Fig. 2.135 Urothelial carcinoma. H&E (high magnification)

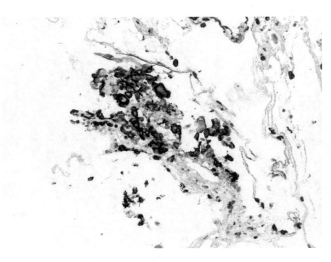

Fig. 2.136 Urothelial carcinoma. CK7 immunostain (high magnification)

(Fig. 2.136), GATA-3 (Fig. 2.137), p63 (Fig. 2.138), uroplakin, and thrombomodulin. Some cells may be CK20 positive.

2.5.14 Clear-Cell Renal Carcinoma Cells

In serous effusion, one can observe small sheets of cohesive neoplastic cells with abundant clear or granular cytoplasm and large oval nuclei with prominent nucleoli (Fig. 2.139). The neoplastic cells express CK8, CK18 (Fig. 2.140), vimentin, CD10, (Fig. 2.141), PAX-2, PAX-8 (Fig. 2.142), and renal cell carcinoma antigen.

2.5.15 Papillary Renal Carcinoma Cells in Serous Effusion

Cytologic samples show complex papillary or multilayered structures of neoplastic cuboidal or columnar cells that have

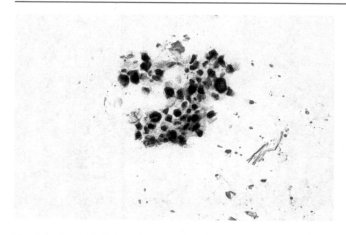

Fig. 2.137 Urothelial carcinoma. GATA-3 immunostain (high magnification)

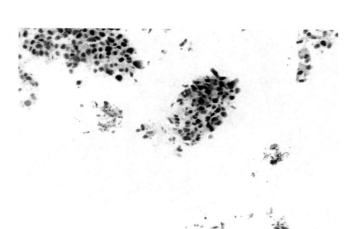

Fig. 2.138 Urothelial carcinoma. p63 immunostain (high magnification)

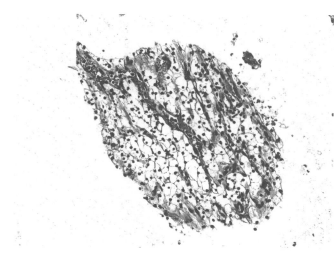

Fig. 2.139 Clear-cell renal carcinoma. H&E (high magnification)

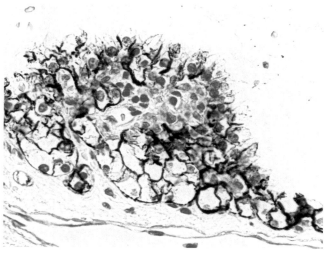

Fig. 2.140 Clear-cell renal carcinoma. CK18 immunostain (high magnification)

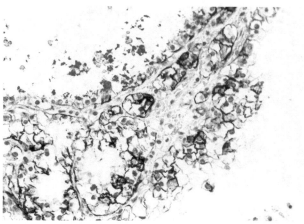

Fig. 2.141 Clear-cell renal carcinoma. CD10 immunostain (high magnification)

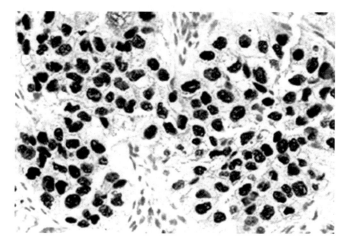

Fig. 2.142 Clear-cell renal carcinoma. PAX-8 immunostain (high magnification)

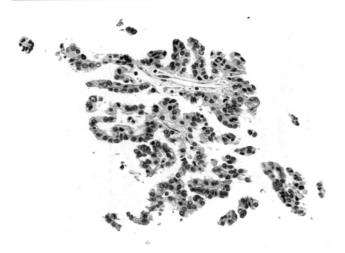

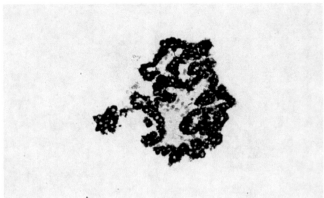

Fig. 2.145   Papillary renal cell carcinoma. AMACR (racemase) immunostain (high magnification)

Fig. 2.143   Papillary renal cell carcinoma. H&E (high magnification)

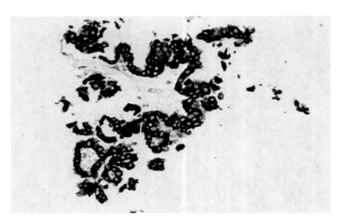

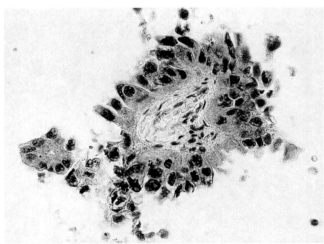

Fig. 2.144   Papillary renal cell carcinoma. CK7 immunostain (high magnification)

Fig. 2.146   Papillary renal cell carcinoma. PAX-2 immunostain (high magnification)

scant pale or granular cytoplasm and round/oval nuclei with prominent nucleoli (Fig. 2.143).

In type I carcinoma, the neoplastic cells show a positive immunoreaction with CK7 (Fig. 2.144), vimentin, CD10, AMACR (Fig. 2.145), PAX-2 (Fig. 2.146), and PAX-8. Negative CK7 is usually seen in the type II variant.

2.5.16   Bellini's Duct Renal Carcinoma Cells in Serous Effusion

In cytologic samples, the neoplastic cells are grouped in a packed cohesive, papillary, or duct-like structure (Fig. 2.147). Morphologically, the neoplastic cells are usually in a columnar shape with granular or vacuolated cytoplasm, large eccentric nuclei, coarse chromatin, and prominent nucleoli. The immunocytochemistry is positive for CK8 (Fig. 2.148),

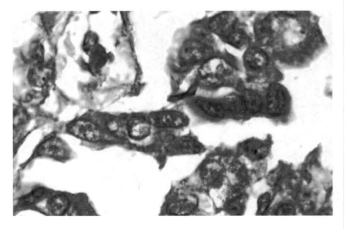

Fig. 2.147   Bellini's duct renal cell carcinoma. H&E (high magnification)

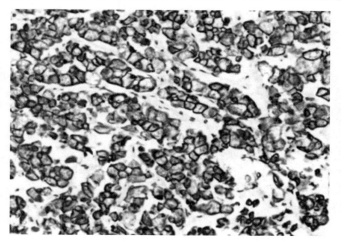

Fig. 2.148 Bellini's duct renal cell carcinoma. CK8 immunostain (high magnification)

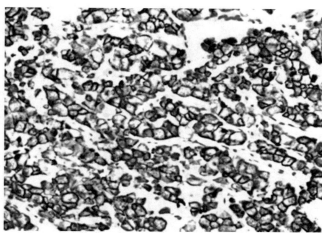

Fig. 2.150 Bellini's duct renal cell carcinoma. CK7 immunostain (high magnification)

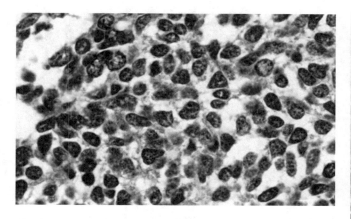

Fig. 2.149 Bellini's duct renal cell carcinoma. PAX-8 immunostain (high magnification)

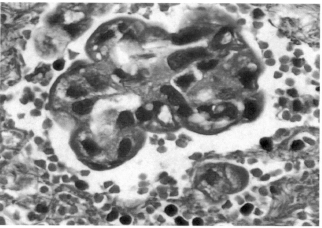

Fig. 2.151 Ductal pancreas cell carcinoma. H&E (high magnification)

CK18, CK19, PAX-8 (Fig. 2.149), and E-cadherin. Focal expression of CK7 (Fig. 2.150), EMA, EpCAM, RCC, CD10, HER-2, and vimentin can be observed. HER-2 usually is hyper-expressed.

2.5.17 Ductal Pancreas Carcinoma Cells in Serous Effusion

In cytologic samples, the neoplastic cells appear pleomorphic, polygonal, cuboidal, or columnar, with delicate, vacuolated, or squamoid cytoplasm that may contain mucin. Nuclei are enlarged and pleomorphic with prominent nucleoli (Fig. 2.151). Neoplastic cells are positive for CK7 (Fig. 2.152), CK17 (Fig. 2.153), and DUPAN-2. Some cells also express CK20 (Fig. 2.154).

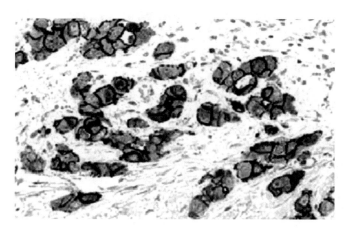

Fig. 2.152 Ductal pancreas cell carcinoma. CK7 immunostain (high magnification)

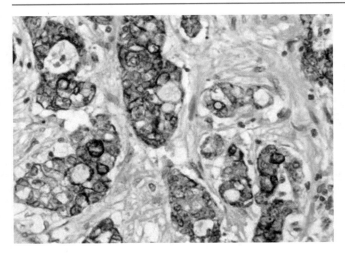

Fig. 2.153　Ductal pancreas cell carcinoma. CK17 immunostain (high magnification)

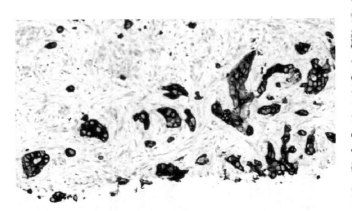

Fig. 2.154　Ductal pancreas cell carcinoma. CK20 immunostain (high magnification)

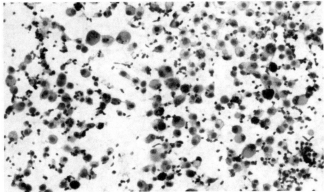

Fig. 2.155　Melanoma cells. Papanicolaou stain (medium magnification)

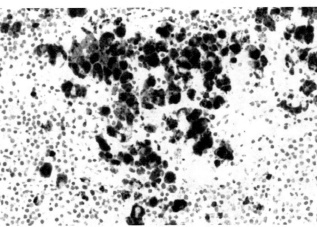

Fig. 2.156　Melanoma cells. Melan A/Mart-1 immunostain (high magnification)

2.5.18　Secondary Lymphohematopoietic Neoplasia Involvement in Serous Effusion

All types of lymphomas and leukemias can involve serous cavities. Lymphoma cells of small-cell type must be differentiated from reactive lymphoid cells and large-cell lymphomas from epithelial and myeloid malignancies. This distinction is usually reached by conventional cytodiagnosis and immunostains. However, when a secondary lymphoproliferative disorder is suspected, flow-cytometric immunophenotyping is the best method for confirming the diagnosis.

2.5.19　Melanoma Cells in Serous Effusion

Neoplastic cells can be observed singly or in cohesive clusters of round, plasmacytoid, pleomorphic, or spindle cells of variable size and scant to large cytoplasm and containing melanin pigment granules in melanotic melanomas. Nuclei

have a regular or anaplastic appearance with macronucleoli and may exhibit intranuclear inclusions (Fig. 2.155).

Immunocytochemistry usually is positive for S-100 protein, Melan A/Mart-1 (Fig. 2.156), HMB-45, SOX-10, and CD63 (NKI/C-3).

2.5.20　Soft Tissue Sarcoma Cells in Serous Effusion

All soft tissue sarcomas that invade serous membranes can exfoliate in serous fluids, even though this is a rare occurrence. Ewing and synovial sarcoma and desmoplastic small-cell tumor are the mesenchymal malignancies that most frequently exfoliate in serous effusions. It is necessary to have clinical data, as well as immunocytochemical and biomolecular investigations, for assessment of the presence of sarcoma cells and for making the correct diagnosis.

Ewing sarcoma cells in serous effusion (Askin tumor) are polygonal with oval nuclei and scant cytoplasm (Fig. 2.157); they are seen singly or forming small rosettes. Immunocytochemistry shows positivity for CD99 (Fig. 2.158), Fli-1, and WT-1 and lacks other mesenchymal markers, whereas molecular genetics shows translocation t(11;22)(q24;q12), t(21;22)(q22;q12), t(7;22)(p22;q12), t(17;22)(q21;q12), or t(2;22)(q33;q12).

Exfoliated synovial sarcoma in serous effusion shows spindle cells in loose clusters with or without epithelium-like cells (Fig. 2.159). Neoplastic cells express vimentin, CD99, bcl-2, calretinin, EMA, and, focally, CK7 and CK19. Recently, the development of TLE-1 (Fig. 2.160) antibody has allowed the detection of the translocation t(X;18)(p11;q11).

In serous effusions (usually peritoneal), desmoplastic small-round-cell tumors show neoplastic cells arranged singly and in clusters. Neoplastic cells are small, usually round, with scant, occasionally vacuolated cytoplasm, and round/oval nuclei have finely granular chromatin and inconspicuous nucleoli (Fig. 2.161). The immunocytochemistry is positive for vimentin,

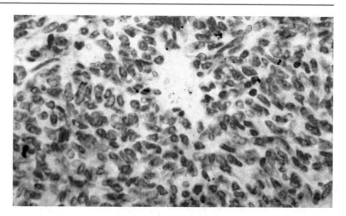

Fig. 2.159 Synovial sarcoma. H&E (high magnification)

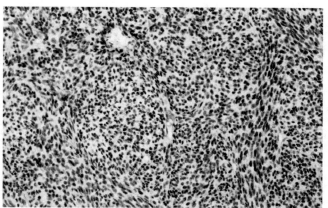

Fig. 2.160 Synovial sarcoma. TLE-1 immunostain (medium magnification)

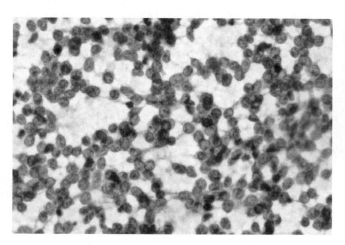

Fig. 2.157 Ewing sarcoma/PNET. Papanicolaou stain (high magnification)

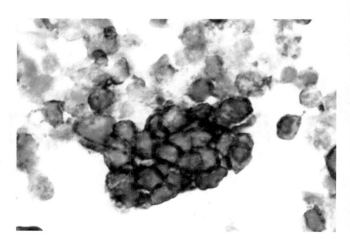

Fig. 2.158 Ewing sarcoma/PNET. CD99 immunostain (high magnification)

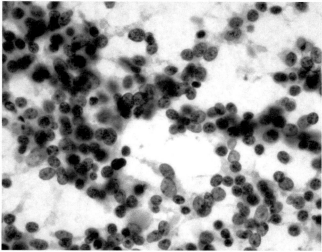

Fig. 2.161 Desmoplastic small round cell tumor. H&E (high magnification)

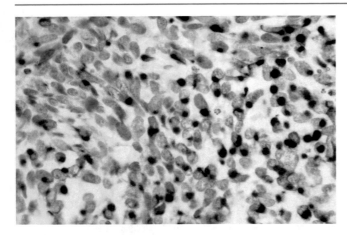

Fig. 2.162 Desmoplastic small round cell tumor. Desmin immunostain (high magnification)

CK8, CK18, EMA, CD99, and WT1. A characteristic feature is the dot-like pattern in desmin immunostaining (Fig. 2.162). Neoplastic cells show a t(11;22)(p13;q12) translocation.

Suggested Reading

Carbone M, et al. Molecular analyses, morphology and immunohistochemistry together differentiate pleural synovial sarcomas from mesotheliomas: clinical implications. Anticancer Res. 2002;22:3443.

Davidson B. The diagnostic and molecular characteristics of malignant mesothelioma and ovarian/peritoneal serous carcinoma. Cytopathology. 2011;22:5.

Grefte JM, et al. Improved identification of malignant cells in serous effusions using a small, robust panel of antibodies on paraffin-embedded cell suspensions. Acta Cytol. 2008;52:35.

Hanna A, et al. Podoplanin is a useful marker for identifying mesothelioma in malignant effusions. Diagn Cytopathol. 2010; 38:262.

Hassan SA. Diagnostic utility of cell blocks and an immunomarker panel in the cytological evaluation of serous effusions. Arch Cytol Histopathology Res. 2019;4:47.

Hasteh F, et al. The use of immunohistochemistry to distinguish reactive mesothelial cells from malignant mesothelioma in cytologic effusions. Cancer Cytopathol. 2010;118:90.

Hyun TS, et al. The diagnostic utility of D2-40, calretinin, CK5/6, desmin and MOC-31 in the differentiation of mesothelioma from adenocarcinoma in pleural effusion cytology. Acta Cytol. 2012; 56:527.

Kato Y, et al. Immunohistochemical detection of GLUT-1 can discriminate between reactive mesothelium and malignant mesothelioma. Mod Pathol. 2007;20:215.

Lozano MD, et al. Immunocytochemistry in the differential diagnosis of serous effusions. Cancer Cytopathol. 2001;93:68.

Oda T, et al. Immunocytochemical utility of claudin-4 versus those of Ber-EP4 and MOC-31 in effusion cytology. Diagn Cytopathol. 2016;44:499.

Pastore C, et al. Distribution of Kaposi's sarcoma herpesvirus sequences among lymphoid malignancies in Italy and Spain. Br J Haematol. 1995;91:918.

Saleh HA, et al. Differentiating reactive mesothelial cells from metastatic adenocarcinoma in serous effusions: the utility of immunocytochemical panel in the differential diagnosis. Diagn Cytopathol. 2009;37:324.

Silverman JF. Effusion cytology of metastatic malignancy of unknown primary. AJSP Rev Rep. 2001;6:154.

Su XY, et al. Cytological differential diagnosis among adenocarcinoma, epithelial mesothelioma, and reactive mesothelial cells in serous effusions by immunocytochemistry. Diagn Cytopathol. 2011;39:900.

Subbarayan D, et al. Use of panel of markers in serous effusion to distinguish reactive mesothelial cells from adenocarcinoma. J Cytol. 2019;36:28.

Sundling KE, et al. Ancillary studies in pleural, pericardial, and peritoneal effusion cytology. Cancer Cytopathol. 2018;126:590.

Exfoliative Cytology

3.1 Respiratory Tract

Exfoliative cytology of the lower respiratory tract can be evaluated in various cytologic samples: deep-coughed sputum, bronchial aspirates, bronchial washing, bronchial brushing, and bronchoalveolar lavage (BAL).

The most frequently obtained sample is sputum. An adequate sample shows variable numbers of squamous cells from the oral cavity and pharynx and scattered alveolar macrophages; cylindrical cells from the trachea and bronchial tree and cuboidal bronchiolar cells are rarely seen.

3.2 Normal Exfoliated Cells

Ciliated columnar and goblet cells are rarely seen in induced sputum samples but are often seen in cytologic specimens obtained after bronchoscopy or in extensive damage of the respiratory epithelium. Numerous ciliated columnar cells can be observed in bronchial washings, aspirates, or brushings. Small cell clusters of bronchial epithelium can be observed in BALs and in transbronchial and transthoracic fine-needle aspiration (FNA) samples. In bronchial brushings, lavage specimens, and aspirates, the respiratory epithelium usually appears as small fragments constituted of uniform columnar ciliated cells, which show a tail-like process at one end and cilia at the opposite (luminal) end. The nuclei are round to oval, with thin chromatin and one or multiple small nucleoli. Ciliated cells express CK7, CK8, CK18, and CK19.

Goblet cells with cytoplasmic mucoid inclusions and flattened, basally placed nuclei can be observed along with ciliated cells. Goblet cells are usually observed in samples from patients who have bronchiectasis, asthma, or chronic bronchitis. These cells can be stained with various antibodies to carbohydrate antigens (CA19.9, B72.4, and others) and MUC5AC.

Bronchial aspirates, bronchial lavages, and, particularly, brushing samples frequently show reserve (basal) cells, whereas these are present only occasionally in sputum, because they do not exfoliate spontaneously. Reserve cells are small, round, or polygonal, with scant cytoplasm, and they show tiny, darkly stained, and homogeneously structured nuclei. Basal cells express CK5 (or CK5/6), CK14, CK17, and p63.

Terminal bronchiolar cells, alveolar pneumocytes, and Kulchitsky cells are very rare or are not present in cytologic samples except in some BALs and FNAs. Normal type 1 pneumocytes are not recognizable in cytologic specimens. Type 2 pneumocytes have a moderate amount of cytoplasm and some intranuclear vacuoles. They express CK7, CK8, CK18, CK19, TTF-1, napsin A, MUC-1, and surfactant.

Kulchitsky cells are a part of the diffuse neuroendocrine system; they occur singly or in very small clusters, admixed with basal cells. Kulchitsky cells are not recognizable in bronchial brushings and aspirates without specific histochemical or immunocytochemical stains. These neuroendocrine cells display chromogranin A, synaptophysin, and CD56 reactivity.

3.3 Infectious Pulmonary Disease

The incidence of lower respiratory tract infections, seen particularly in immunocompromised patients, has increased. The use of immunocytochemistry allows identification of the microbiological infective agent(s) previously diagnosed by conventional microscopy and histochemical stains.

Bacterial Infections Usually, immunocytochemistry is not used for determination of the specific types of bacterial organisms in cytological specimens. A molecular biology PCR test for identifying mycobacterial infection can be applied to lower respiratory tract samples, including BAL obtained from patients with a clinical suspicion of tubercular infection, which often shows necrotic debris, as well as epithelioid and multinucleated histiocytes.

© Springer Nature Switzerland AG 2020
E. Leonardo, R. H. Bardales, *Practical Immunocytochemistry in Diagnostic Cytology*,
https://doi.org/10.1007/978-3-030-46656-5_3

Viral Infections Viral pneumopathies are common in immunosuppressed patients. The most frequent viral agents are herpes viruses such as cytomegalovirus (CMV), herpes simplex (HSV), herpes zoster (HZV), as well as measles and adenovirus. CMV infection show enlarged bronchial cells and pneumocytes with large intranuclear inclusions (Fig. 3.1). Cytoplasmic inclusions can be seen in some cases. In difficult cases, positive anti-CMV immunostaining (Fig. 3.2) confirms the presence of CMV infection.

Clustered epithelial and multinucleated cells with ground-glass nuclei and intranuclear inclusions, usually eosinophilic (Fig. 3.3), characterize the exfoliative cytology of a herpetic infection. The diagnosis can be confirmed by specific antibody immunocytochemistry reactions (Fig. 3.4).

Measles and respiratory syncytial virus (RSV) infections yield similar cytologic findings in exfoliative lung cytology. In fact, giant multinucleated epithelial cells with eosinophilic cytoplasmic and intranuclear inclusions can be observed (Fig. 3.5). The use of specific antibody immunostains allows the characterization of the viral agent (Fig. 3.6).

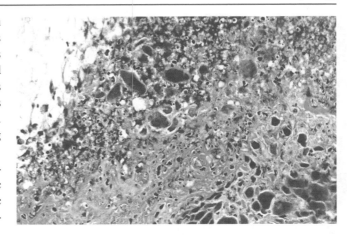

Fig. 3.3 Epithelial cells with herpetic infection (high magnification)

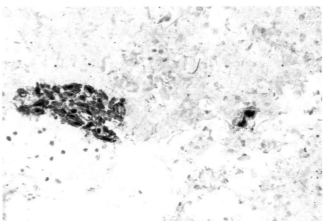

Fig. 3.4 Anti-HSV immunostain positive cells (high magnification)

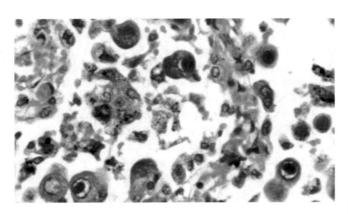

Fig. 3.1 CMV infected cells. H&E (high magnification)

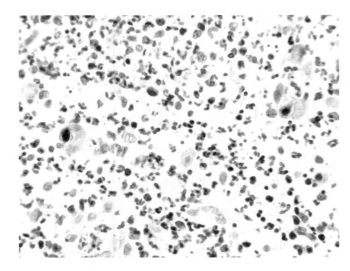

Fig. 3.2 Anti-CMV immunostain positive cells (high magnification)

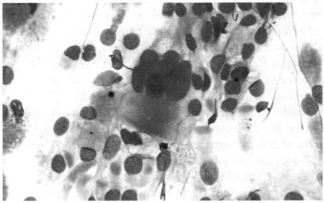

Fig. 3.5 RSV infection (high magnification)

An adenovirus-infected bronchial epithelium is characterized by the presence of cells with large smudgy nuclei, which have multiple small inclusions (Fig. 3.7) or a single small eosinophilic intranuclear inclusion. Adenovirus infection is often associated with ciliocytophthoria. A spe-

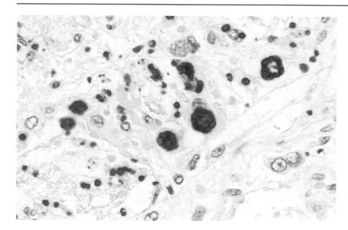

Fig. 3.6 Anti-RSV positive cells immunostain (high magnification)

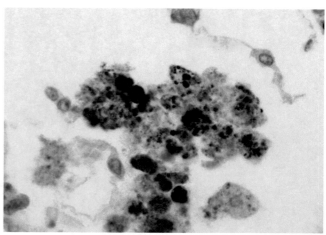

Fig. 3.8 Anti-adenovirus immunostain positive cells (high magnification)

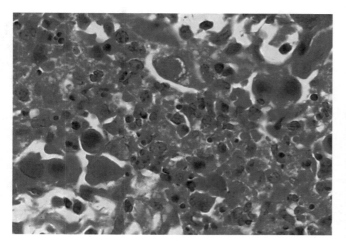

Fig. 3.7 Adenovirus infection (high magnification)

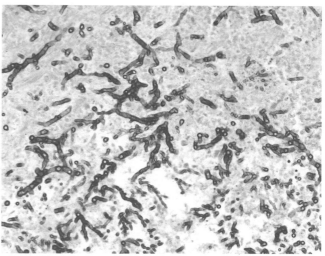

Fig. 3.9 Aspergillosis H&E (high magnification)

cific type of immunostaining can be used for confirming the presence of adenovirus (Fig. 3.8).

Fungal Infections Various types of fungi (*Blastomyces, Cryptococcus neoformans, Histoplasma capsulatum, Coccidioides immitis, Candida albicans, Aspergillus niger, Pneumocystis jirovecii*) can cause pulmonary infections in immunocompromised patients. Particularly frequent infections are pneumopathies due to *Candida*, *Aspergillus*, and *Pneumocystis*. These organisms can be demonstrated by cytomorphology and histochemistry stains (PAS reaction, Gomori silver methenamine) in BAL material, bronchial washings, and induced sputum samples.

In cytology samples, *Candida* appears in the form of pseudo hyphae and clusters of yeasts. The presence of only yeast forms in sputum may be considered to be due to oral contamination.

Aspergillus has septate hyphae with a constant diameter (3–6 μm), parallel edges, and dichotomous branching at acute angles (Fig. 3.9). This organism can form a fungus ball (asper-

gilloma) with fruiting heads (conidiophores). Birefringent calcium oxalate crystals seen under polarized light may be recognized in *Aspergillus niger* infections (Fig. 3.10). Immunocytochemistry sometimes is carried out for differentiation of aspergillosis (Fig. 3.11) from other, similar mycoses.

Pneumocystis jirovecii, formerly known from the name of a protozoon, *Pneumocystis carinii*, causes alveolar foamy exudates or casts with organisms that appear as tiny bubbles or vacuoles. The cysts represented by the vacuoles inside the alveolar casts are spherical, oval, or cupped structures with a flat surface and measure from 5 to 7 μm in the maximum dimension. Inside the cysts, there are one or two dot-like trophozoites or sporozoites that measure 0.5 to 1 μm in diameter (Fig. 3.12). The presence of *Pneumocystis jirovecii* can be detected by immunostains with the use of a specific antibody (Fig. 3.13).

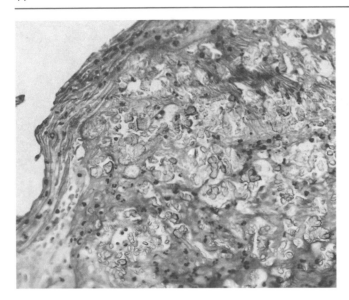

Fig. 3.10 Aspergillosis calcium oxalate crystals H&E (high magnification)

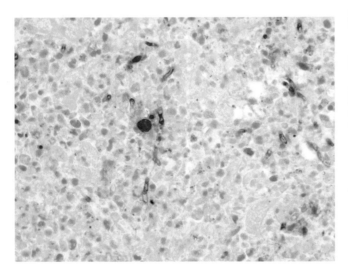

Fig. 3.11 Anti-*Aspergillus* immunostain (high magnification)

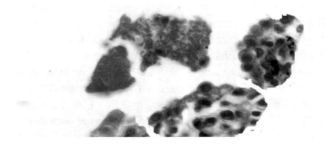

Fig. 3.12 *Pneumocystis jirovecii* H&E (high magnification)

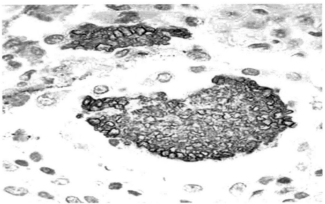

Fig. 3.13 Anti-*Pneumocystis* immunostain (high magnification)

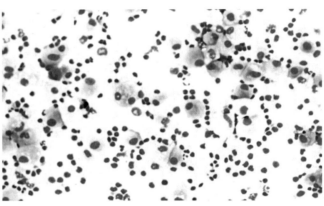

Fig. 3.14 Sarcoidosis, BAL. Romanowsky stain (high magnification)

3.4   Noninfectious Pulmonary Disease

Sarcoidosis Cytology shows numerous lymphocytes, giant multinucleated cells, and epithelioid histiocytes (Fig. 3.14). Occasionally, the giant cells can contain intracytoplasmic star-shaped crystals (asteroid bodies) and small lamellar calcified bodies (Schaumann bodies). Rare granulocytes are observed. Necrosis may be present in rare cases. Immunocytochemistry highlights the presence of predominantly CD4-positive T cells (Fig. 3.15) and rare CD8-positive lymphocytes (Fig. 3.16), with an abnormal CD4/CD8 ratio, usually 4–6:1.

Extramedullary Hematopoiesis This can occur in patients with chronic hemolytic conditions such as thalassemia, sickle cell anemia, hereditary red blood cell disease, erythroblastosis fetalis, and polycythemia vera. Moreover, it can develop when the bone marrow is replaced by leukemia, lymphoma, or metastatic carcinoma. Immunocytochemistry with CD34, CD117, TdT, and pan-CK helps to differentiate between extramedullary hematopoiesis and extramedullary myeloid tumor.

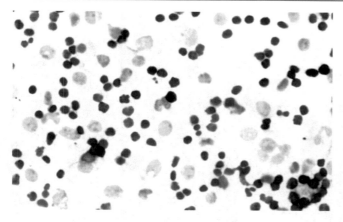

Fig. 3.15 Sarcoidosis, BAL, CD4 immunostain (high magnification)

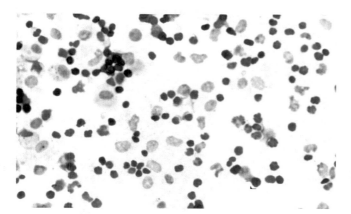

Fig. 3.16 Sarcoidosis, BAL, CD8 immunostain (high magnification)

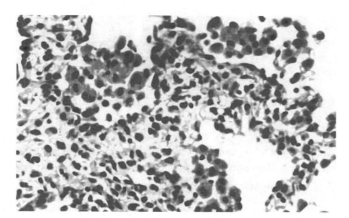

Fig. 3.17 Langerhans cell. Romanowsky stain (high magnification)

Langerhans Cell Histiocytosis An inflammatory background composed of eosinophils, lymphocytes, histiocytes, and neutrophils is seen in BAL and bronchial washings. The Langerhans cells (Fig. 3.17) show ample eosinophilic cytoplasm, which contains Birbeck granules on electron microscopy. Nuclei are irregular with prominent folds and grooves; the chromatin is fine with indistinct nucleoli. These cells

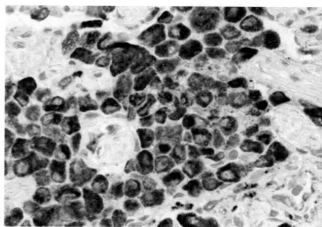

Fig. 3.18 Langerhans cells, CD1a immunostain (high magnification)

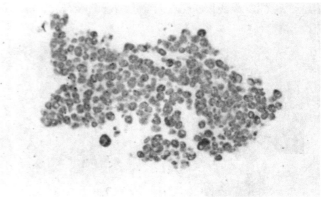

Fig. 3.19 Langerhans cell, Langerin immunostain (high magnification)

express S100 protein, CD1a (Fig. 3.18), and CD207 (langerin) (Fig. 3.19). Positivity for CD68 is variable, and some cells can show mutations of the *BRAF* oncogene as demonstrated by BRAF positive immunostaining.

3.5 Primary Lung Cancer

Squamous Cell Carcinoma In sputum samples, squamous cell carcinoma in situ usually shows single round or oval small cells, frequently with keratinized cytoplasm, hyperchromatic nuclei, and sometimes small nucleoli; however, no tumor necrosis is seen. It is worth emphasizing that malignant squamous cells in sputum may be derived not only from endobronchial sites but may also originate in the oral cavity, pharynx, larynx, or trachea. Moreover, it is not possible to differentiate squamous cell carcinoma in situ from the invasive form on a purely cytologic basis.

Invasive squamous cell carcinomas usually exfoliate large numbers of neoplastic cells into the sputum, washings, or brushings. Variable amounts of necrosis are seen in the smear background. Well-differentiated cancer cells appear singly and in loose clusters, with irregular cytoplasmic keratinization, nuclear pleomorphism with irregular coarse chromatin, and no visible nucleoli. Keratin pearls may be observed. Poorly differentiated squamous cell carcinoma shows a mixture of single pleomorphic cells and minute complex aggregates of neoplastic cells (Fig. 3.20).

Immunocytochemistry allows the identification of the squamous nature of poorly differentiated cells that show positive immunostaining for p40 (Fig. 3.21) and desmocollin-3 (Fig. 3.22). Neoplastic cells also show CK5 (Fig. 3.23) or CK/6 positivity, but the WHO considers this marker not to be a determinant for assessing the squamous cell nature of lung cancer. The squamous cell marker p63 is less specific than p40, because it can be positive in 30% of lung adenocarcinomas. TTF-1, napsin A, and neuroendocrine markers are negative. CK7 occasionally can stain some poorly differenti-

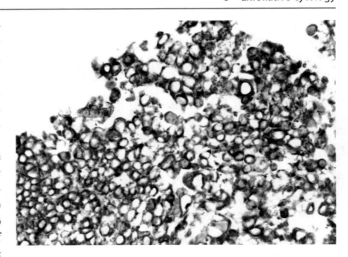

Fig. 3.22 Squamous cell carcinoma, desmocollin-3 immunostain (high magnification)

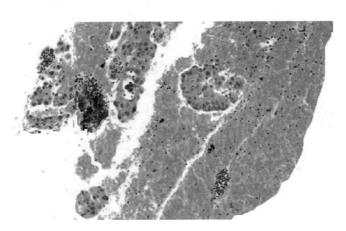

Fig. 3.20 Squamous cell carcinoma. H&E (high magnification)

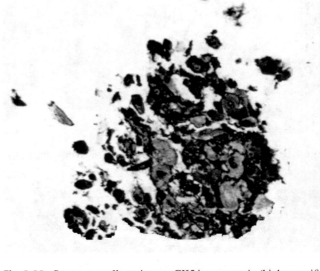

Fig. 3.23 Squamous cell carcinoma, CK5 immunostain (high magnification)

ated neoplastic squamous cells. Cytologic samples can be used for determining the presence of the PD-L1 marker (Fig. 3.24) on neoplastic cells.

Adenocarcinoma This tumor is usually situated peripherally in the lung; therefore, it may show a small number of cells or no cells at all in exfoliative cytology samples. The exfoliation mainly depends on the tumor site and tumor size. Cytologically, single cells and small cell aggregates with ball-like, acinar, or papillary architecture may be observed. Neoplastic cells have a homogeneous, foamy, or vacuolated cytoplasm producing margination of the nucleus. Usually, the nuclei are eccentric or lobulated, with dispersed or granular chromatin and evident nucleoli (Fig. 3.25).

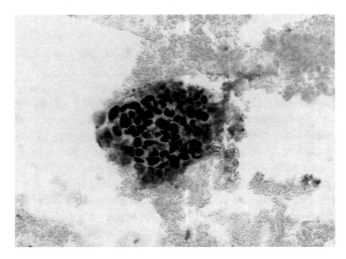

Fig. 3.21 Squamous cell carcinoma, p40 immunostain (high magnification)

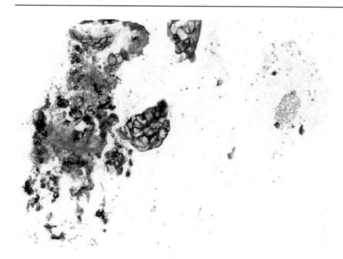

Fig. 3.24 Squamous cell carcinoma, PDL-1 immunostain (high magnification)

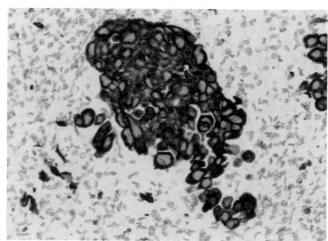

Fig. 3.26 Adenocarcinoma, CK7 immunostain (high magnification)

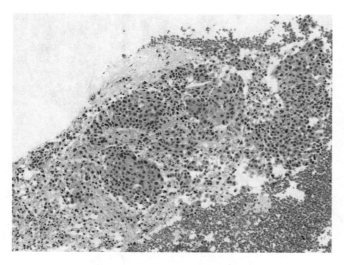

Fig. 3.25 Adenocarcinoma. H&E (high magnification)

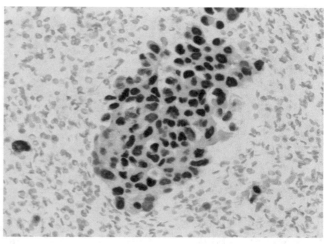

Fig. 3.27 Adenocarcinoma, TTF-1 immunostain (high magnification)

Lung adenocarcinoma cells are positive for CK7 (Fig. 3.26), TTF-1 (Fig. 3.27), napsin A (Fig. 3.28), sometimes for surfactant proteins, and for CEA, B72.3, ESA, and ERA markers. Neuroendocrine and squamous cell markers are negative, except for p63, which may be positive in up to 30% of cases. Evaluation for markers useful in determination of personalized oncology therapy, such as ALK (Fig. 3.29) and ROS-1 (Fig. 3.30), can be carried out on cytologic specimens.

Neuroendocrine Tumors These neoplasms are distributed in the proximal parts of the lung. They are often found in the bronchial submucosa and are covered by normal respiratory epithelium. Thus, sputum cytology is often negative, whereas it is possible to find the neoplastic cells in brushing samples.

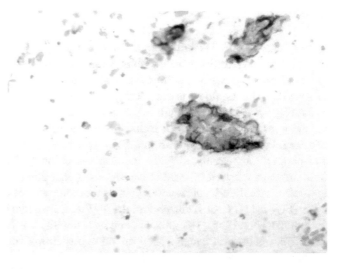

Fig. 3.28 Adenocarcinoma, napsin A immunostain (high magnification)

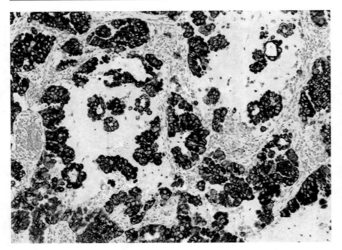

Fig. 3.29 Adenocarcinoma, ALK immunostain (high magnification)

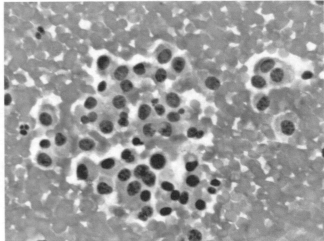

Fig. 3.31 Typical carcinoid. Romanowsky stain (high magnification)

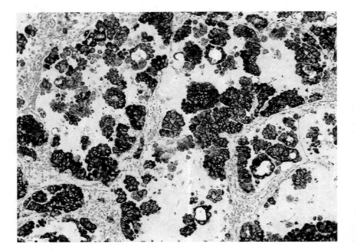

Fig. 3.30 Adenocarcinoma, ROS-1 immunostain (high magnification)

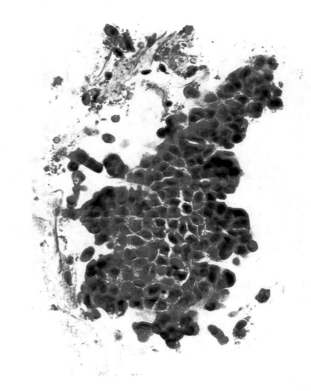

Fig. 3.32 Atypical carcinoid. Romanowsky stain (high magnification)

In typical (Fig. 3.31) and atypical carcinoids (Fig. 3.32), the cytology preparations usually show single cells or small clusters, sometimes small solid nests, trabeculae, papillae, or rosettes. The single cells are usually round or cuboidal, and rarely spindle-shaped, with moderate or limited granular cytoplasm. The nuclei are round or oval with smooth and regular membranes; chromatin is speckled ("salt-and-pepper" appearance), with inconspicuous nucleoli. Sometimes, a mesh of branching capillaries is encountered in a cell-block slide. Typical and atypical carcinoids express CK8 (Fig. 3.33), CK18, chromogranin A (Fig. 3.34), synaptophysin (Fig. 3.35), NSE, CD56, and occasionally CK7. A dot-like pattern is usually seen on immunostaining for cytokeratins. Atypical carcinoid differs from typical carcinoid; only the former shows necrotic cells, and they differ in their proliferation index. The MIB-1 (Ki67)-positive

neoplastic cells in typical carcinoid amount to less than 3% (Fig. 3.36), whereas in atypical carcinoid (Fig. 3.37), the positivity is between 5% and 20%. Moreover, atypical carcinoid usually expresses CK19, and about 25–30% of them are positive for TTF-1.

Small-cell neuroendocrine carcinoma (NEC) smears show bare nuclei and loosely aggregated and dispersed cells which are very fragile, often showing pressure/crush artifact (Fig. 3.38). When well-preserved, above all in brushing samples, the neoplastic cells are small or intermediate in size,

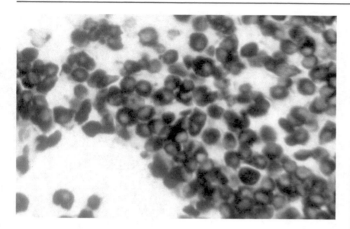

Fig. 3.33 Typical carcinoid, CK8 immunostain (high magnification)

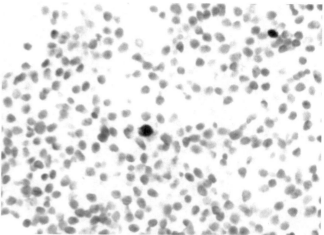

Fig. 3.36 Typical carcinoid, MIB-1 immunostain (high magnification)

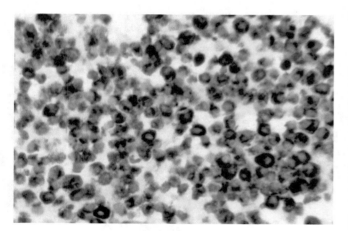

Fig. 3.34 Typical carcinoid, chromogranin A immunostain (high magnification)

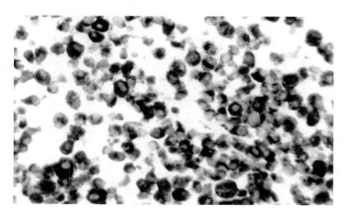

Fig. 3.35 Typical carcinoid, synaptophysin immunostain (high magnification)

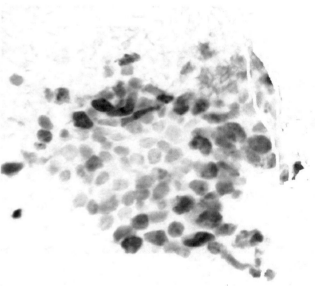

Fig. 3.37 Atypical carcinoid, MIB-1 immunostain (high magnification)

immunostaining pattern. The percentage of MIB-1 (Ki67) immunoreactive cells amounts to more than 25% (Fig. 3.42).

Large-cell neuroendocrine carcinoma (LCNEC) shows more abundant cytoplasm than does NEC, similar nuclear and chromatin features but prominent nucleoli resembling non-small-cell carcinoma (poorly differentiated adenocarcinoma or squamous cell carcinoma). A diagnosis of LCNEC requires positive immunostaining for synaptophysin, chromogranin A, and CD56.

Large-Cell Carcinoma According to the WHO classification, the diagnosis of "large-cell carcinoma" is restricted

with scant cytoplasm and round or oval nuclei that have fine chromatin and inconspicuous nucleoli. NEC shows positivity for CK8, CK18, CK19 (Fig. 3.39), chromogranin A, synaptophysin (Fig. 3.40), NSE, TTF-1 (Fig. 3.41), CD56, and occasionally CK7. Cytokeratin stain usually shows a dot-like

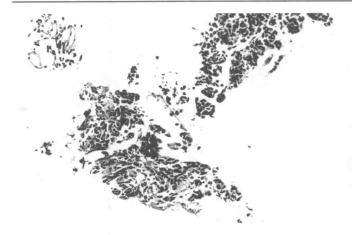

Fig. 3.38 Neuroendocrine small-cell carcinoma. H&E (high magnification)

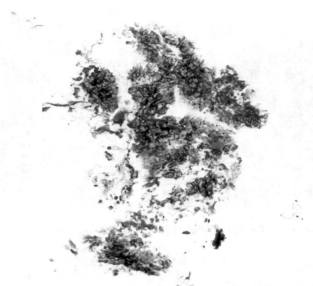

Fig. 3.40 Neuroendocrine small-cell carcinoma. Synaptophysin immunostain (high magnification)

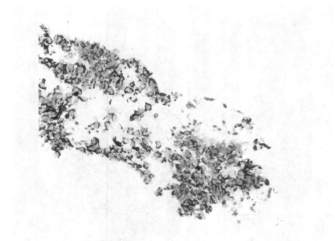

Fig. 3.39 Neuroendocrine small-cell carcinoma. CK19 immunostain (high magnification)

exclusively to histologic resection specimens, whereas in cytopathology the term "non-small-cell carcinoma" can be used when the tumor shows no squamous, glandular, or neuroendocrine differentiations and there is no way of further refining the diagnosis. The neoplastic cells exfoliated in sputum, bronchial washings, and brushings are single or form small clusters, with syncytial arrangements, multinucleation, or giant-cell features. The cytologic diagnosis of malignant neoplasia is straightforward, but the precise diagnosis of this tumor is suspected only if immunocytochemistry was used (see Table 3.1).

Large-cell carcinoma with rhabdoid features has large cytoplasmic globules. However, it does not represent a specific subtype of large-cell carcinoma but rather a cytologic morphologic variant. Also, clear-cell carcinoma, composed of large polygonal cells with abundant clear cytoplasm, does not constitute a specific subtype. The immunophenotype

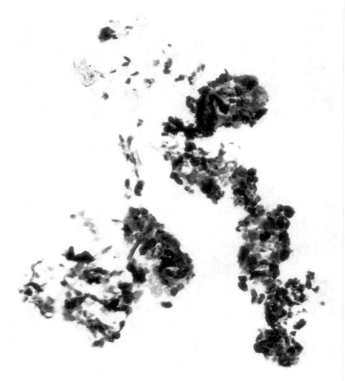

Fig. 3.41 Neuroendocrine small-cell carcinoma. TTF-1 immunostain (high magnification)

seen in large-cell and clear-cell carcinomas is similar to that of other undifferentiated large-cell carcinomas.

Sarcomatoid Carcinoma This carcinoma includes pleomorphic carcinoma, spindle cell carcinoma, giant-cell carci-

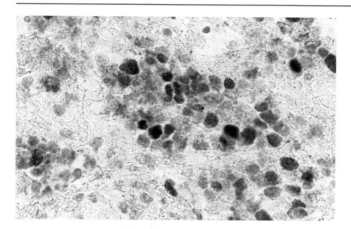

Fig. 3.42 Neuroendocrine small-cell carcinoma. MIB-1 immunostain (high magnification)

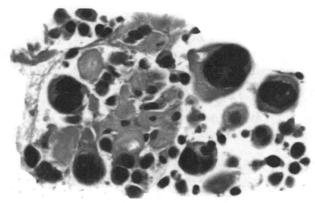

Fig. 3.43 Giant-cell carcinoma. H&E (high magnification)

Table 3.1 Immunocytochemistry of large-cell carcinoma

TTF-1	Napsin A	p40	p63	CK5 or CK5/6	CK7	Diagnosis
+	+ or −	−	−	−	+ or −	Favor adenocarcinoma
−	+	−	−	−	+ or −	Favor adenocarcinoma
+	+ or −	−	+	−	+ or −	Favor adenocarcinoma
+	+ or −	−	+ or −	Focal +	+ or −	Favor adenocarcinoma
−	−	+	+ or −	+	+ or −	Favor squamous cell carcinoma
−	−	−	+ or −	−	+ or −	Large-cell carcinoma, NOS
+	+ or −	+	+	+	+	Might be adenosquamous carcinoma

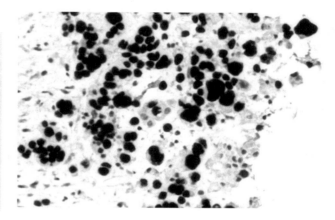

Fig. 3.44 Giant-cell carcinoma, TTF-1 immunostain (high magnification)

noma, carcinosarcoma, and pulmonary blastoma. Most tumors are located peripherally, and the neoplastic cells are rarely observed in exfoliative cytology samples; however, when cells are present, cytological preparations show single and loosely clustered, bizarre malignant cells. Pleomorphic carcinoma consists of cells of various sizes, variable amounts of cytoplasm, and single or multiple, large irregular nuclei with prominent nucleoli. Large malignant spindle cells with hyperchromatic nuclei can be present. Spindle cell carcinoma is composed of a mixture of spindle cells with irregular nuclei and relatively abundant cytoplasm, as well as large malignant cells. Giant-cell carcinomas show enormous neoplastic polygonal cells with a single nucleus or lobulated or multiple nuclei; neutrophilic emperipolesis by tumor giant cells can be seen (Fig. 3.43). Every effort must be made to narrow the morphologic diagnosis of these tumors, looking for squamous or adenocarcinoma markers by use of immunocytochemistry.

Immunocytochemistry shows no sarcomatoid differentiation but does show variable expression of epithelial antigens. Three different situations may arise: (1) some neoplastic cells show positive adenocarcinoma markers (CK7, TTF-1, and/or napsin A), foci of cells positive for squamous markers (CK5 or CL5/6, p40, and/or desmocollin-3), and, sometimes, some cells of neuroendocrine type; (2) all neoplastic cells express only an adenocarcinoma immunophenotype, such as TTF-1 (Fig. 3.44) and/or napsin A; and (3) all neoplastic cells express only squamous-cell antigens.

Pulmonary blastoma and carcinosarcoma are true biphasic neoplasms, as they are composed of neoplastic epithelial and mesenchymal cells. Pulmonary blastoma has an epithelial component of cuboidal and columnar cells with frequently found cytoplasmic vacuoles containing glycogen, and a spindle cell component of mesenchymal (myxoid, chondroid, osteoid, rhabdomyoblastic) cells. Squamoid morules are sometimes present. The epithelial component of this neoplasia stains diffusely with antibodies to epithelial markers, such as CK7, CK8, CK18, CK19, CEA, and epithelial membrane antigen. Some morular and glandular cells may be positive for chromogranin A, synaptophysin, TTF-1, surfactant, and Clara cell protein. Occasionally, some cells are also positive for some hormones, such as calcitonin, bombesin, leu-enkephalin, and somatostatin. The mesenchymal elements are positive for vimentin and, depending on the type of differentiation, for S100 protein, desmin, or myoglobin.

Carcinosarcoma has a carcinoma component admixed with sarcomatous spindle cells. Neoplastic epithelial cells can be of any histotype, but squamous cell carcinoma is the most common. The sarcomatous component may be constituted of neoplastic elements with cartilage, bone, or skeletal muscle differentiation.

Lymphoepithelioma-Like Carcinoma This rare neoplasia usually is located peripherally in the lung; therefore, it is rarely seen in exfoliative cytology specimens. The neoplastic cells are usually large with a syncytial appearance, with round or oval vesicular nuclei, prominent nucleoli, and finely granular to flocculent cytoplasm. There is a lymphocytic infiltrate in the background, and occasionally a spindle cell growth and mitotic figures may be seen.

Immunocytochemical stain shows the squamous cell immunophenotype with positivity for CK5 (or CK5/6), p40 (Fig. 3.45), p63, desmocollin-3, protein kinase C, and EBV-encoded RNA (EBER) (Fig. 3.46). The interspersed lymphocytes are predominantly T cells with cytotoxic characteristics.

NUT Midline Carcinoma Here, the neoplastic cells are loosely cohesive and isolated, with scant cytoplasm and indistinct cell borders. The nuclei are hyperchromatic, round to oval with slightly irregular contours, and with finely granular chromatin containing one or more prominent nucleoli (Fig. 3.47).

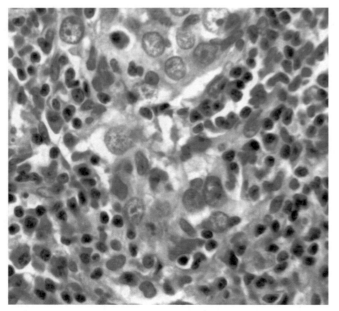

Fig. 3.45 Lymphoepithelioma-like carcinoma. H&E (high magnification)

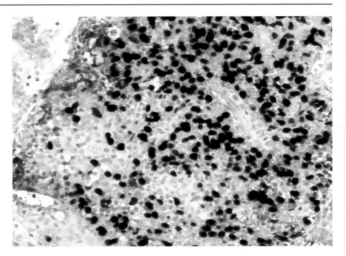

Fig. 3.46 Lymphoepithelioma-like carcinoma, EBER (high magnification)

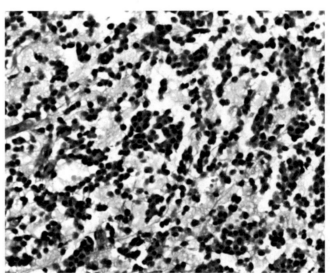

Fig. 3.47 NUT midline carcinoma. H&E (high magnification)

The immunohistochemical profile is characterized by positivity to the NUT protein (Fig. 3.48), expression of the translocation of the *NUT* gene (*NUTM1*) to the *BRD3*, *BRD4*, or *NSD3* gene. Usually, the neoplastic cells are positive for p63, whereas they are variably positive for other lung cancer markers. Immunostaining for CK5 (or CK5/6), CK7, TTF-1, CD99, chromogranin A, and synaptophysin can be observed focally either in single cells or in most of the neoplastic cells.

Adenoid Cystic Carcinoma The neoplastic epithelial cells are bland-appearing and uniform, with scant cytoplasm and dark, round, or oval nuclei. Cellular clusters are surrounded by a hyaline, basement membrane-like substance that is immunopositive for collagen IV and laminin. The tumor

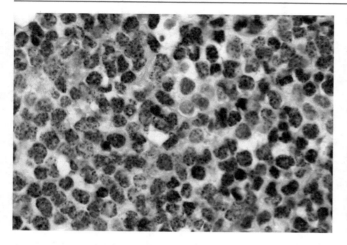

Fig. 3.48 NUT midline carcinoma, NUT protein immunostain (high magnification)

cells show positive staining for CK7, CK8, CK18, CK19, p63, smooth muscle actin, calponin, and S100 protein. Some cells express CK5, CK14, and CK17.

Mucoepidermoid Carcinoma This malignancy usually arises peripherally in the lung; thus, neoplastic cells are rarely seen in exfoliative cytology specimens. Cytologic material shows an admixture of neoplastic squamoid cells and mucin-containing tumor cells together with variable amounts of extracellular mucus. Low-grade mucoepidermoid carcinoma is composed of a monotonous tumor cell population with squamous and glandular differentiation, whereas high-grade tumors show poorly differentiated cells, mostly of the nonkeratinizing squamous type, and scant glandular differentiation. The neoplastic cells are positive for CK5, CK7, CK8, CK14, CK17, CK18, CK19, and EMA. A positive cytoplasmic immunostain for MUC-2, MUC-4, and MUC-5AC is also observed in the neoplastic cells.

3.6 Non-epithelial Lung Tumors

Hematologic Neoplasias Various types of leukemias and Hodgkin and non-Hodgkin lymphomas can involve the lung as part of a systemic disease. Most primary lung lymphomas are marginal-zone B-cell lymphoma of mucosa-associated lymphoid tissue (MALToma), diffuse large B-cell lymphoma, or lymphomatoid granulomatosis.

MALToma is a lymphoma composed predominantly of small lymphocytes. Its diagnosis needs flow cytometry or an adequate cell block for assessment of B-cell monoclonality.

Primary pulmonary diffuse large B-cell lymphomas exhibit a monomorphous population of large lymphocytes with one to three nucleoli. Flow cytometry or cell-block sec-

tions are required for determining the expression of B-cell antigens and a monoclonal B-cell population.

The diagnosis of lymphomatoid granulomatosis cannot be made on cytologic specimens, because abundant tissue is needed morphologically for verifying the presence of an angiocentric clonal lymphoid proliferation and for determining the amount of EBV-positive large B-cells.

Soft Tissue Tumors Primary benign and malignant soft tissue tumors of the lung are exceedingly rare in exfoliative cytology specimens. Sarcomas are usually metastatic, and their cytologic diagnoses are made on samples usually obtained by image-guided fine needle aspiration.

3.7 Biliary Tract

For benign and malignant processes involving the biliary tract, the method for the collection of ductal cells includes brushings during cholangiographic studies, washings of the bile canaliculi, aspiration of pure bile from the bile ducts, direct collection of secreted bile, endobiliary brush cytology during percutaneous transhepatic cholangio-drainage, and aspiration of duodenal secretions.

Normal Extrahepatic Biliary Tract Cells Normal epithelial cells of the large biliary ducts appear slender, tall, and columnar with abundant thin, sometimes finely vacuolated cytoplasm, and basally placed small, round to oval nuclei with dispersed fine chromatin and small or inconspicuous nucleoli. Mixed with the columnar cells, there are some cuboidal epithelial cells. The epithelial cells are positive for CK7, CK8, CK18, and CK19; some cells also express CK20.

Reactive Cells Reactive cytologic changes occur in lithiasis, acute sclerosing cholangitis, and infections, among other non-neoplastic conditions. Inflammation causes loss of cellular surface structure, and the cells show some vacuolization of the cytoplasm, minimal nuclear enlargement, hyperchromasia with granular, evenly dispersed chromatin, and conspicuous single or multiple nucleoli. Some cells with mucinous or squamous metaplasia can be observed. The inflamed epithelial cells show the same immunophenotype as that of normal cells. Positivity for MUC5AC and MUC-6 is also present.

Intraepithelial neoplasia (Dysplasia) Cellular changes increase as the grade of dysplasia progresses. In low-grade forms, sheets and groups of cells with nuclear crowding and overlapping are observed. Nuclei are slightly enlarged and have smooth membranes. In high-grade dysplasia, three-dimensional complex cell groups with cellular overlap are present. The nuclei are enlarged and show nuclear membrane irregularity and coarse chromatin. The distinction of high-grade dysplasia from carcinoma in situ cannot be made with certainty on a purely cytologic basis. Dysplastic cells are positive for CK7, CK8, CK18, CK19, MUC-1, MUC-2, and MUC5AC.

Intraductal Papillary Mucinous Neoplasm The degree of cellular abnormalities depends on the grade of the dysplasia seen in this neoplasm. The cytologic features of papillary differentiation include papillary formations of crowded and overlapping groups of cells. The atypical mucinous cells present in biliary brushings are columnar with abundant cytoplasmic mucin, nuclear atypia, and subtle irregularities of the nuclear membrane and nucleoli. Neoplastic cells express CK7, CK8, CK18, CK19, CD15, CD117, CD34, DOG1, MUC-1, and MUC5AC.

Adenoma The adenomatous epithelium consists of thin and elongated columnar cells arranged singly or in small sheets and clusters. The cells show oval, basally oriented nuclei that occupy about a third of the cell body. The nuclei have fine granular chromatin and one or more nucleoli. Tumor cells display positivity for CK7, CK8, CK19, villin, and CA antigens. Some cells show apical positivity for CD10 and CD56.

Bile Duct Adenocarcinoma The neoplasia of the distal bile ducts is similar to that of the proximal perihilar type. An increased number of mucin-producing cells and focal intestinal epithelial differentiation, including goblet cells and endocrine cells, can be observed. Loosely cohesive cell clusters, disorganized sheets, dense cell clusters showing acinar-like or micropapillary features, and pleomorphic cells are observed in variable numbers (Fig. 3.49). Nuclear overlapping, a pronounced loss of polarity, nuclear membrane irregularities, in particular wrinkling and molding, and prominent irregularly

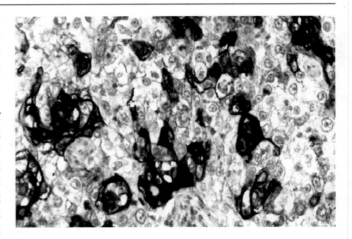

Fig. 3.50 Bile duct adenocarcinoma. CK7 immunostain (high magnification)

shaped nucleoli can be present. Neoplastic epithelial cells show CK7 (Fig. 3.50), CK8, CK18, and CK19. Variable numbers of tumor cells express CK20, EMA, CEA, MUC-2, CD15, and p53. Mucin-producing cells may have positivity for MUC5AC, CA19–9, CDX-2, and TAG-72 (B72.3).

Ampullary Adenocarcinoma Ampullary adenocarcinoma and bile duct adenocarcinoma are morphologically similar, although ampullary neoplasms appear more like primary adenocarcinomas of the intestinal tract, and they may have a predominant villous or papillary pattern. Exfoliative cytology samples show a variable complex papillary architecture and papillary fronds. Furthermore, pseudostratified columnar cells are observed, with overlapping polymorphic nuclei.

Neoplastic cells have positive immunocytochemical stains for CK8, CK18, CK19, CK20, MUC-2, CDX2, CEA, and CA19–9. Some tumor cells express CK7 and DUPAN-2.

3.8 Pancreatic Tract

Cytologic material is obtained by intraductal brushing and aspiration of the cells exfoliated from pancreatic ducts by use of endoscopic retrograde cholangiopancreatography. Other, less frequently used methods of investigating possible pancreatic lesions are examination of the cells in the pancreatic juice including direct aspiration, washing of the duct system, suction after secretin stimulation, or fluid collection from the orifice of the ampulla of Vater.

Normal Pancreatic Exfoliated Cells Acinar cells usually are arranged in small- to medium-sized cohesive groups, sometimes with a central lumen. Single and grouped cells appear triangular or pyramidal, having abundant finely granular cytoplasm and round, eccentric, or central nuclei with

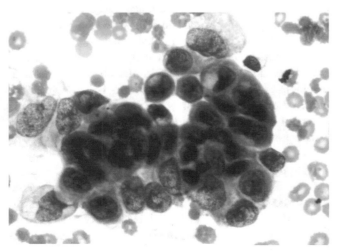

Fig. 3.49 Bile duct adenocarcinoma, H&E (high magnification)

fine granular chromatin and small distinct nucleoli. Acinar cells are immunopositive for CK8, CK18, bcl-10, and trypsin. Some cells express CK7, CK19, PDX-1, and glyplican-3.

Epithelial cells lining large pancreatic ducts are seen in sheets forming palisades or in regular flat, honeycomb-like structures. Cells are small to medium sized, cuboidal to columnar, with scant, sometimes vacuolated cytoplasm. Nuclei are small, round, and exhibit dispersed and fine granular chromatin with an occasional tiny nucleolus. Normal pancreatic duct cells are positive for CK7, CK8, CK18, CK19, MUC1, MUC6, CA19–9, MOC31, PSCA, mesothelin, annexin A8, pVHL, DPC4/SMAD4, and claudin 4 and 18.

Islet cells are rarely found in normal pancreatic aspirates. When present, these cells appear in minute, vaguely cohesive aggregates; they are round to oval with pale or flimsy cytoplasm, central or eccentric round nuclei, and finely granular chromatin. Islet cells are positive for the general endocrine immunostaining markers, chromogranin A, synaptophysin, neuron-specific enolase, and Leu7. Moreover they are positive for CK8, CK18, PSCA, IMP-3, pVHL, MOC31, DPC4/SMAD4, and claudin 4 and 18.

Ductal Pancreatic Adenocarcinoma Here, hypercellular samples are usually observed, in which ductal cells predominate in a clean, inflammatory, mucinous, or necrotic background. The neoplastic ductal cells are arranged in sheets or in complex overcrowded and/or disorderly groups (Fig. 3.51). Variable numbers of atypical isolated cells are also present. The neoplastic cells show a well-defined cytoplasmic border, and enlarged atypical nuclei with irregular contours, coarse chromatin, and macronucleoli. The different degrees of nuclear pleomorphism, anaplasia, and bi- and multinucleation have a direct relationship to the degree of tumor differentiation.

There are different variants of ductal pancreatic adenocarcinoma. Large, bizarre, multinucleated giant cells and/or pleomorphic spindle-shaped cells can be observed in the anaplastic variant. Neoplastic bizarre, spindle-shaped to epithelioid mononuclear cells and non-neoplastic multinucleated osteoclastic-like giant cells are seen in the osteoclastic giant-cell tumor variant. Neoplastic cells with large cytoplasmic vacuoles that push the atypical nuclei to the periphery are typically seen in the signet-ring cell variant. The foamy-gland variant is composed of cells with abundant foamy cytoplasm, basally located hyperchromatic nuclei, and an apical brush border-like cytoplasmic condensation.

Regardless of the cytomorphologic variant, the neoplastic cells express CK7, CK8, CK18, CK19, maspin, S100 protein, IMP-3 (Fig. 3.52), MOC31, DUPAN-2, annexin A8, and claudin 4 (Fig. 3.53) and 18. Positive cells for CEA, CEACAM-1, CD44v6, PSCA, mesothelin, CA19.9, MUC-

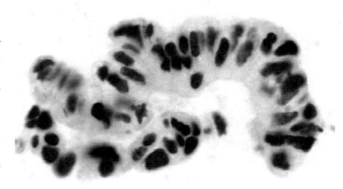

Fig. 3.52 Ductal pancreatic adenocarcinoma, IMP-3 immunostain (high magnification)

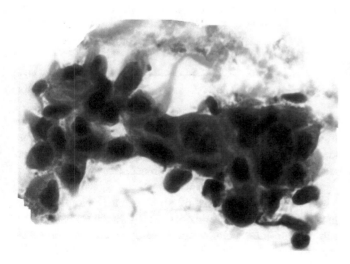

Fig. 3.51 Ductal pancreatic adenocarcinoma, H&E (high magnification)

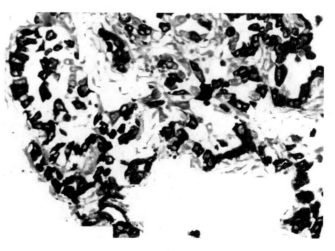

Fig. 3.53 Ductal pancreatic adenocarcinoma, claudin-4 immunostain (high magnification)

1, MUC-4, and MUC5AC can be present. Some neoplastic cells also express CK20 and/or CK17. Neoplastic cells are negative for DPC4/SMAD4.

Acinar Cell Carcinoma Cytologic aspirates of this carcinoma are usually highly cellular and are composed of numerous single cells and loosely cohesive cell aggregates, sometimes showing variable acinar formations (Fig. 3.54). The neoplastic cells have abundant granular cytoplasm with indistinct cytoplasmic borders and central or eccentric nuclei with irregular contours, clumped chromatin, and a single prominent nucleolus. The cytoplasm is fragile and ruptures easily, resulting in the presence of fine granularity in the smear background.

The neoplastic cells are positive for CK8 (Fig. 3.55), CK18, bcl-10, trypsin, chymotrypsin protein (Fig. 3.56),

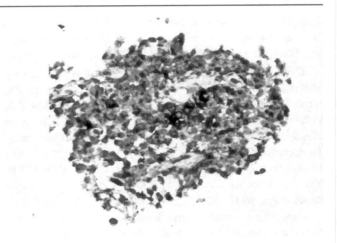

Fig. 3.56 Acinar cell pancreatic adenocarcinoma, chymotrypsin immunostain (high magnification)

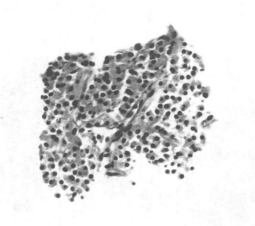

Fig. 3.54 Acinar cell pancreatic adenocarcinoma, H&E (high magnification)

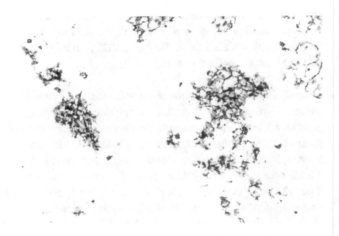

Fig. 3.57 Acinar cell pancreatic adenocarcinoma, E-cadherin immunostain (low magnification)

claudin 7, E-cadherin protein (Fig. 3.57), and PSTI (pancreatic secretory trypsin inhibitor). Some cells can express CK7, EMA, CEA, B72.3, CD44 (Fig. 3.58), MUC5AC, CA19–9, CA125, DUPAN-2, and synaptophysin.

3.9   Urinary Tract

Urine cytology is very sensitive and specific for identification of high-grade urothelial carcinoma, whereas there is known difficulty in recognizing low-grade urothelial cancer cells because of the similarity to reactive urothelial cells or aggregated normal cells of washings.

Cytology preparations of spontaneously voided urine usually show rare single urothelial cells. In contrast, washing samples are more cellular and have characteristic cell clusters. Multinucleated urothelial cells are observed mainly in bladder washing specimens. Urothelial cells present in upper urinary tract washings are similar to those present in urinary

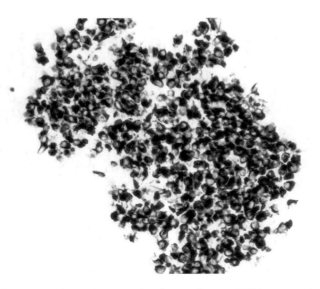

Fig. 3.55 Acinar cell pancreatic adenocarcinoma, CK8 immunostain (high magnification)

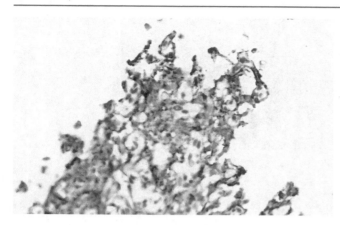

Fig. 3.58 Acinar cell pancreatic adenocarcinoma, CD44 immunostain (high magnification)

bladder washings; however, variable numbers of columnar urothelial cells may be present.

Normal Urothelial Cells Superficial urothelial cells appear single or arranged in loose or cohesive groups of different sizes. They show a wide and dense cytoplasm and bland nuclei with fine granular chromatin and inconspicuous nucleoli. Binucleated cells can be seen. Immunocytochemistry is positive for CK7, CK8, CK18, CK19, and CK20.

Intermediate and basal urothelial cells are usually arranged in regular, compact three-dimensional clusters. These cells are smaller than superficial cells and have a pyramidal or round shape with thin cytoplasm, well-defined cytoplasmic borders, and a single dense nucleus. Some elongated and columnar cells with a fusiform or columnar shape can be observed; they can originate from the urothelial intermediate zone, metaplastic glandular epithelium, periurethral glands, or prostatic epithelium. These cells have a clear cytoplasm with sharp borders. The nuclei have granular and thinly dispersed chromatin, irregular nuclear borders, and variably prominent nucleoli. Intermediate and basal urothelial cells usually express CK7, CK8, CK13, CK18, CK19, and rarely CK4, CK5, CK6, CK13, CK15, and CK17.

Renal epithelial cells are rarely present in urinary specimens. They are difficult to identify, except if they are numerous and appear together with renal casts.

Cell degeneration and Reactive and Reparative Changes Urothelial cells usually show varying degrees of cellular changes and degeneration in inflammatory and infectious processes. According to the Paris classification, all of these cellular changes must be considered benign, i.e., negative for urothelial malignancy. The cellular alterations included in this section concern urine specimens with cellular changes associated with urolithiasis, infections of various types, chemotherapy, and radiotherapy.

Degenerating and reactive/reparative urothelial cells can be distinguished from dysplastic/malignant cells. Sometimes, spindle and columnar urothelial cells may be present in three-dimensional arrangements, simulating a papillary urothelial carcinoma; however, the absence of a fibrovascular core supports the diagnosis of a reactive process.

Urolithiasis The urine sample is usually hypercellular and shows three-dimensional aggregates and papillary fragments without fibrovascular cores. Cells show minimal cytologic atypia, smooth borders, centrally placed enlarged nuclei, and finely granular chromatin. The presence of blood, crystals, and the above-mentioned cellular changes are of help for distinguishing urolithiasis from low-grade papillary urothelial carcinoma.

Urinary Tract Infection In urinary tract *tuberculosis*, epithelioid giant cells (Langhans type) in a background of caseous necrosis can be observed. Alcohol-resistant acid-fast bacilli can be identified by immunohistochemistry; however, immune reactions have low sensitivity and limited specificity for mycobacteria. Polymerase chain reaction test yields more accurate results.

Iatrogenic infection caused by intravesical *bacillus Calmette-Guerin* therapy can produce epithelioid granulomas and granular debris that are seen in urine cytology.

In immunosuppressed patients, especially after transplant, urothelial cells with the characteristic nuclear inclusion of *cytomegalovirus* can be present in urinary specimens. Immunocytochemistry with a specific antibody validates the cytomorphologic diagnosis.

Herpes simplex virus (HSV) infection occasionally can involve bladder urothelial cells, which appear as clusters of multinucleated cells with ground-glass-appearing nuclei and intranuclear inclusions (Fig. 3.59). The presence of HSV-infected cells can be highlighted by use of specific immunoreactions (Fig. 3.60).

Polyoma virus infection produces nuclear enlargement with chromatin homogenization and margination caused by the typical intranuclear viral inclusion (Fig. 3.61). Immunopositive reaction with anti-polyoma virus (SV40, JC, and BK) antibody confirms the viral infection (Fig. 3.62).

Cellular changes caused by urethral *papilloma virus* (HPV) infection, i.e., koilocytosis, can be encountered occasionally in urine specimens (Fig. 3.63). The use of anti-p16 immunoreactions allows identification of the high-risk HPV-infected cells (Fig. 3.64).

Chemotherapy Effect Chemotherapy and immunosuppressive drugs cause degenerative or reactive urothelial cell changes. Reactive urothelial cells are characterized by the presence of coarsely vacuolated cytoplasm, enlarged and sometimes hyperchromatic nuclei, and prominent nucleoli.

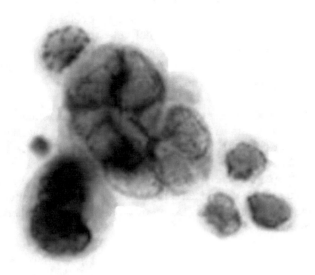

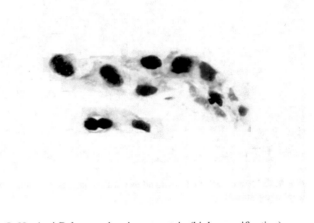

Fig. 3.62 Anti-Polyoma virus immunostain (high magnification)

Fig. 3.59 Herpesvirus urine infected cells, Papanicolaou stain (high magnification)

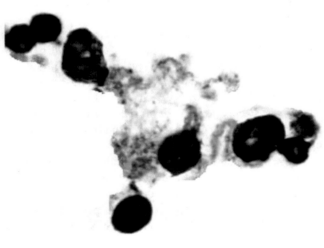

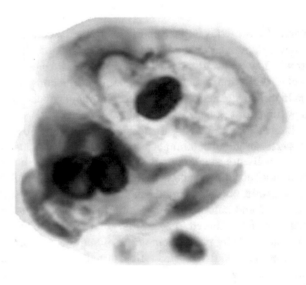

Fig. 3.63 HPV urine infected cells, Papanicolaou stain (high magnification)

Fig. 3.60 Anti-HSV immunostain (high magnification)

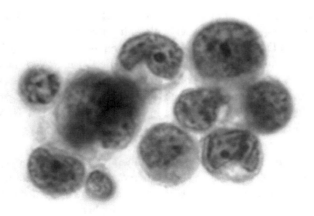

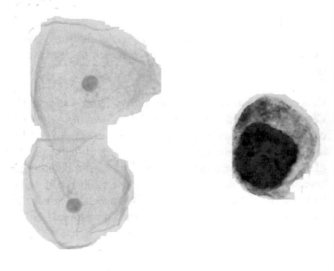

Fig. 3.61 Polyoma virus urine infected cells, Papanicolaou stain (high magnification)

Fig. 3.64 Anti-p16 immunostain (high magnification)

Radiotherapy After radiotherapy, urothelial cells appear enlarged with vacuolated cytoplasm and large nuclei with a normal nuclear-to-cytoplasm ratio. Sometimes the cells are multinucleated.

Atypical (Dysplastic) Urothelial Cells In mild dysplasia, urothelial cells may appear slightly enlarged, sometimes crowded and elongated, with nuclear grooves, nuclear membrane irregularities, finely granular chromatin, and small nucleoli. These changes are similar to those in reactive urothelial cells; therefore, a conclusive diagnosis based on cytomorphologic features alone is often difficult or impossible to make. Moreover, cytometry analysis or routine molecular and immunocytochemical assays cannot differentiate among a benign reactive cell population, a dysplastic cell population, and a low-grade urothelial neoplasm.

In moderate dysplasia, the cells are enlarged, crowded, and frequently elongated, but the overall pattern is uniform. Nuclei show mild hyperchromasia, as well as slightly irregular borders and grooves; the chromatin is dense and grossly granular; nucleoli are small, but distinctly visible. It may be extremely difficult to distinguish moderately dysplastic cells from those of a true urothelial carcinoma or severe reactive/reparative change.

Various biological markers have been proposed for identifying the real neoplastic nature of urothelial cells, but the results obtained do not appear to be conclusive. FISH tests for assessment of the presence of polysomy or deletions can help one to diagnose dysplastic cells. The FISH test (UroVysion®) to look for the polysomy of chromosomes 3, 7, and 17 and deletion of 9p21 can be used for the partial identification of neoplastic urothelial cells. However, it must be remembered that polysomy is observed mainly in high-grade urothelial carcinomas, whereas it is not seen in low-grade ones. Furthermore, the 9p21 deletion occurs in about half the cases of low-grade urothelial carcinoma. The nuclear positivity of the immune reaction with the MCM-2 (minichromosome maintenance 2) antibody is observed in most high-grade urothelial cancer cells but also in atypical cells or polyoma virus infection. Notably, the specificity of MCM-5 immunostaining is not affected by benign proliferative or inflammatory conditions, including bacillus Calmette-Guerin-induced granulomatous cystitis. An immunocytochemical cocktail containing antibodies against TOP2A (topoisomerase IIα) and MCM-2 proteins, known as ProEx C, exhibits high sensitivity in detecting high-grade urothelial carcinoma and low sensitivity in the low-grade form. Recently, the use of CK17 immunostaining has been suggested for distinguishing neoplastic from reactive urothelial cells, because positive staining is rarely seen in the normal and reactive urothelial mucosa. ImmunoCyt/uCyt+ is another immunocytochemical test for identifying urothelial cancer cells. It makes use of three different fluorescent-labeled antibodies directed against a high-molecular-weight form of glycosylated carcinoembryonic antigen, as well as mucins.

High-grade carcinoma cells are enlarged, rounded, or elongated, with hyperchromatic and polymorphous nuclei (Fig. 3.65). The chromatin is granular and coarse, and large pleomorphic nucleoli are present. Cellular groups show a marked loss of polarity. Cells with these features may be seen in either carcinoma in situ (CIS) or invasive urothelial carcinoma. The use of CK20, CD44, p53, and Ki67 has been proposed for distinguishing between CIS and invasive carcinoma cells. Positivity for CK20 and p53 (Fig. 3.66), with a high Ki67 proliferative index and absence of CD44 is seen CIS. The absence of CK20 (although some cells may be positive) and CD44 with p53 positivity would instead be indicative of a high-grade urothelial carcinoma (Fig. 3.67).

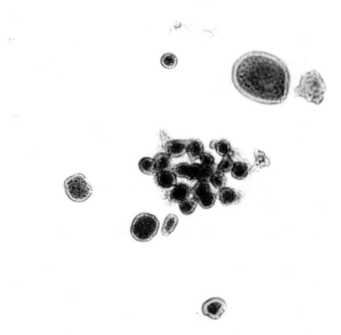

Fig. 3.65 High-grade dysplastic urothelial cell. Papanicolaou stain (high magnification)

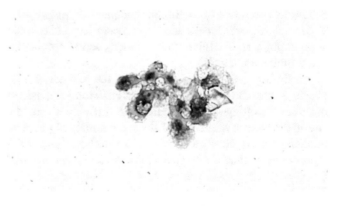

Fig. 3.66 High-grade dysplastic urothelial cell. CK20 (red) and p53 (brown) immunostain (high magnification).

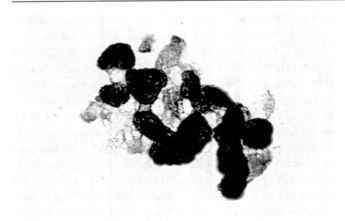

Fig. 3.67 High-grade dysplastic urothelial cell. CD44 (red) and p53 (brown) immunostain (high magnification).

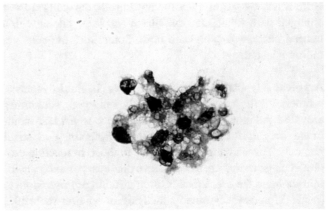

Fig. 3.68 Urothelial CIS. CK20 (red) and p53 (brown) immunostain (high magnification)

Low-Grade Urothelial Neoplasia Low-grade urothelial carcinoma and papillary urothelial neoplasm of low malignant potential are included in this group. In cytologic preparations, urothelial cells can be observed forming groups and pseudo-papillae; however, only those with fibrovascular cores are diagnostic for low-grade neoplasia. Cytologically, the neoplastic cells show a homogeneous cytoplasm, an increased nuclear-to-cytoplasm ratio, and irregular nuclear outlines. However, these characteristics are not sufficient for a conclusive diagnosis.

Some ancillary tests as mentioned above can be used for differentiating cells with similar cytomorphology.

High-Grade Urothelial Neoplasia This category includes CIS and invasive urothelial carcinoma. CIS is associated with marked cell exfoliation and is composed of single, round, or polygonal neoplastic cells with densely structured cytoplasmic borders; focal cytoplasmic vacuolization may be present. Nuclei are hyperchromatic, wrinkled, and folded, with clumped, coarsely granular chromatin and large nucleoli. There is a high nuclear-to-cytoplasm ratio.

Invasive high-grade urothelial carcinoma shows increased cellularity composed of single cells and papillary aggregates. The neoplastic cells have a dense cytoplasm, hyperchromatic pleomorphic nuclei with irregular borders, coarse chromatin, and prominent nucleoli.

According to the Paris classification, the number of neoplastic urothelial cells is an important criterion for classifying urine cytology specimens into the "suspicious" or the "positive" category. In cases of limited numbers of neoplastic cells that are compatible with urothelial carcinoma, the report must be that of "suspicious for urothelial carcinoma." Conversely, if there are more than 10 neoplastic cells, the diagnosis can be urothelial carcinoma.

As mentioned before, CIS shows immunopositivity for CK20 and p53 (Fig. 3.68), whereas CD44 is negative. High-grade invasive urothelial carcinoma is positive for p53, CD44 is negative, and CK20 can be expressed in a few cells. A high percentage of Ki67-positive cells can be observed in both CIS and high-grade invasive urothelial carcinoma.

Squamous Cell Carcinoma Primary pure squamous cell carcinoma is very rare and is observed mainly in areas of Africa where it is strongly associated with *Schistosoma haematobium* infections. In contrast, cells with squamous differentiation can be observed frequently in cases of high-grade urothelial carcinoma. The presence of a large number of neoplastic squamous cells in urine samples from female patients can be suggestive of cervical cancer spreading into the urinary bladder, an important consideration in the differential diagnosis.

Urothelial Adenocarcinoma This is also a rare neoplasm, which is usually related to urachal remnants. Smears of well-differentiated adenocarcinoma show isolated columnar cells with amphiphilic, finely vacuolated cytoplasm, hyperchromatic nuclei, and glandular formations. In poorly differentiated carcinomas, signet-ring cells and high-grade malignant cells with prominent nucleoli are seen (Fig. 3.69).

Neoplastic cells express CK7 (Fig. 3.70), CK8, CK18, CK19, and CD141. Some CK20- and CDX-2-positive cells can be observed.

Neuroendocrine Carcinoma This is also known as small-cell carcinoma and has a cytomorphology similar to that seen in smears from other sites, i.e., small, round to oval cells with scant cytoplasm, hyperchromatic nuclei with "salt-and-pepper" chromatin, and nuclear molding. Neoplastic cells express chromogranin A, synaptophysin, CD 56, and sometimes TTF-1.

Metastatic Carcinoma Renal carcinomas rarely exfoliate neoplastic cells into the urine. Therefore, it is difficult to

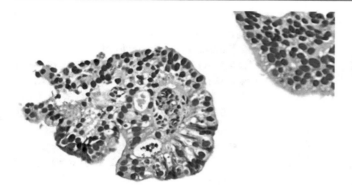

Fig. 3.69 Bladder adenocarcinoma, H&E (high magnification)

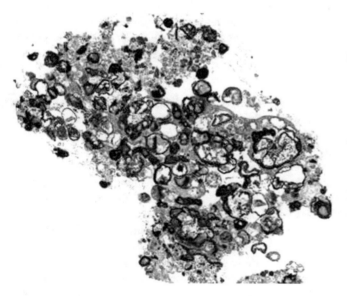

Fig. 3.70 Bladder adenocarcinoma, CK7 immunostain (high magnification)

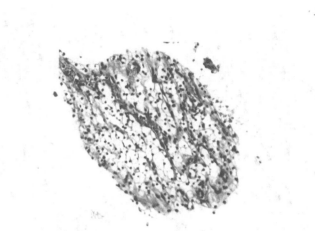

Fig. 3.71 Clear cell renal cell carcinoma, H&E (high magnification)

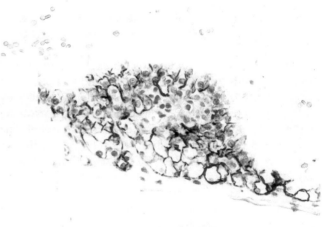

Fig. 3.72 Clear cell renal cell carcinoma, CD10 immunostain (high magnification)

make a cytologic diagnosis on urine preparations. When exfoliation occurs, the exfoliated renal cancer cells are mostly of the clear-cell type. They show an abundant, foamy, and vacuolated cytoplasm; therefore, it is necessary to distinguish these cells from activated histiocytes, bladder clear-cell carcinoma cells, and nephrogenic adenoma cells (Fig. 3.71). The use of immunostaining for renal cell carcinoma, i.e., RCC marker, CD10 (Fig. 3.72), PAX2, and PAX8, with absence of p63 and GATA-3, supports the diagnosis of metastatic renal cell carcinoma.

Exfoliated prostatic carcinoma cells in urine specimens almost always occur in patients with high-grade, unresectable tumors. The presence of prostate cancer is already known clinically in most cases, whereas its presence is suggested by urine cytology only in rare cases in which the history is unknown. In some cases, cells have relatively abundant cytoplasm and round nuclei with prominent nucleoli (Fig. 3.73); in other cases, cells have features similar to those of urothelial cells. Positive immunocytochemistry for

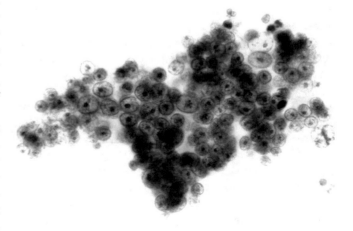

Fig. 3.73 Prostate cancer cells, Papanicolaou stain (high magnification)

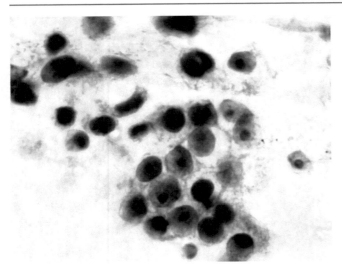

Fig. 3.74 Prostate cancer cell. NKX3 immunostain (high magnification)

prostate-specific membrane antigen (PSMA), prostein (p501S), and NKX3 (Fig. 3.74) can help one identify prostate cancer cells.

Colonic carcinoma can involve the bladder neck; therefore, cancer cells can exfoliate and be found in urine specimens. Distinction from urothelial carcinoma is usually difficult, because the neoplastic cells appear pleomorphic with degenerated, hyperchromatic, and irregular nuclei. The immunophenotype of metastatic colon cancer cells is characteristic: positivity for CK20 and CDX-2, with negative immunostaining for CK7.

3.10   Female Genital Tract

Ectocervical and endocervical cells can be collected after exfoliation induced by various brush systems, such as the Ayre spatula or the endocervical broom. The exfoliated cells can be smeared directly onto a slide (conventional Pap) or placed in a liquid-based cytology medium. Spontaneously exfoliated endometrial cells can also be found in cervical cytology samples; however, endometrial cells can also be harvested by means of direct endometrial brushing.

Normal Exfoliated Cells Ectocervical squamous superficial and intermediate cells are large and polygonal. Superficial cells have a small pyknotic nucleus, whereas intermediate cells show nuclei with finely granular chromatin and are occasionally binucleated. Parabasal cells are round or oval and have a variably sized nucleus but one that is larger than that of an intermediate cell. Basal cells, which are rarely found in cervical samples, are smaller than parabasal cells and have very scant cytoplasm. Superficial cells express CK4, CK6, CK13, and occasionally CK1, CK10,

and CK11. Most intermediate cells can be immunostained with CK4, CK6, and CK13 and only some with CK10, CK11, and CK14. Parabasal cells have immunoreactivity for CK6, CK13, CK14, CK18, and CK19, whereas only some cells can be marked with CK4 and CK5. Basal cells express CK5, CK6, CK14, CK18, CK19, and EGF-R, with occasional positivity for CK8.

Endocervical cells are columnar, with abundant vacuolated cytoplasm and an eccentric nucleus with a finely granular chromatin texture. Endocervical cells are positive for CK7, CK8, CK18, and CK19 and some also for CK5, CK13, and CK14.

Exfoliated endometrial cells are usually arranged in spherical clusters and can be seen during menstrual bleeding and up to 12 days thereafter. They are small, with scant cytoplasm and dark nuclei. Endometrial cells express CK7, CK8, CK18, and CK19, as well as estrogen and progesterone receptors.

Cell degeneration and Reactive and Reparative Changes Various conditions may cause normal squamous and endocervical cells to exhibit features that mimic malignancy.

Nuclear enlargement and mild hyperchromasia are usually observed in intermediate squamous cells during perimenopause. In endocervical inflammation, endocervical polyps, and pregnancy (Arias-Stella reaction), columnar cells are large with abundant cytoplasm and enlarged round or oval nuclei, usually with a large nucleolus. The immunophenotype of these cells is that of the normal cells.

Reparative changes follow the healing process of traumatic lesions of the cervical squamous epithelium, and reserve cells re-epithelialize the areas of epithelial damage. A typical repair cytology pattern includes cohesive flat sheets of enlarged, uniform cells, with an enlarged nucleus and prominent nucleolus.

Radiation produces acute and chronic cellular alterations that can last for a long period of time. Cells are enlarged, isolated, or in groups and show cytoplasmic vacuolization and polychromasia, enlarged nuclei, and finely granular chromatin. Similar changes can be induced by chemotherapy. Immunocytochemistry highlights the normal antigen expression.

An intrauterine device (IUD) might cause a dense inflammatory response and reactive cytologic changes due to mechanical effects that cause local irritation. Two different cellular patterns can be observed in cytologic samples: (1) large glandular cells arranged singly or in small clusters, showing abundant vacuolated cytoplasm that may displace the enlarged nucleus with a visible nucleolus to the periphery of the cell, and (2) cells with scant cytoplasm, irregular chromatin, and a large nucleus (IUD cells), which can be confused with cells of intraepithelial neoplasia. In this case, the positivity of the immunoreaction for anti-p16 protein allows differentiating these changes from those in HPV-infected cells.

Infectious processes Other than HPV *Trichomonas vaginalis* infection produces a nonspecific small, narrow, indistinct perinuclear halo in the squamous cells, accompanied by minimal nuclear atypia. The parasitic protozoan organism can be identified by a specific antibody, whereas the squamous cells show a normal immunophenotype.

In fungal infection by *Candida albicans* and *Candida glabrata*, there is a minimally reactive cellular change, and some squamous cells have a small perinuclear halo. Immunocytochemistry does not contribute to the diagnosis.

Herpes simplex virus (HSV) infection is characterized by typical nuclear features that include a "ground-glass" appearance, thick nuclear membranes, and sometimes eosinophilic intranuclear inclusions. Multinucleation with nuclear molding is common. Positivity with the specific HSV antibody confirms the infection.

Cytomegalovirus (CMV)-infected cells are stromal and/or endocervical in origin. They are enlarged and have multiple small, granular cytoplasmic inclusions and a solitary nuclear basophilic inclusion surrounded by a halo. Occasionally, intermediate squamous cells show granular cytoplasmic inclusions. The presence of CMV infection can be highlighted with a specific CMV immunostaining.

Chlamydia trachomatis involves endocervical and/or metaplastic cells and exhibits intracytoplasmic vacuoles that usually contain central, small coccoid bodies. The infected cells show non-specific nuclear enlargement and slight hyperchromasia. Multinucleation may be seen. Immunocytochemistry can identify the presence of *Chlamydia*.

HPV infections are discussed in the section on squamous cell abnormalities as they are related to cervical malignancies.

HPV-Related Squamous Cell Abnormalities *Human papilloma virus* (HPV) infection causes "koilocytosis," the characteristic cytopathic effect seen in cervical squamous cells (Fig. 3.75). Cells show cytoplasmic cavitation with a rim of condensed cytoplasm, nuclear enlargement with coarse chromatin, and irregular nuclear membranes. The rim of condensed cytoplasm, which gives the cell a clear appearance, surrounds the eccentrically placed dysplastic nucleus. The presence of these cells is indicative of HPV infection.

Low-grade squamous intraepithelial lesion (LSIL) is a lesion of superficial and/or intermediate cells in which one can observe moderate nuclear enlargement with slight nuclear membrane irregularities and variable anisonucleosis. Some cells show binucleation, smudgy hyperchromasia, and inconspicuous nucleoli.

High-grade squamous intraepithelial lesion (HSIL) consists of immature squamous cells, single or arranged in cohe-

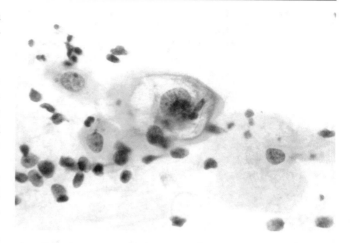

Fig. 3.75 Koilocyte cells, Papanicolaou stain (high magnification)

sive groups, with indistinct cell borders (syncytium-like clusters). Hyperchromasia, an irregular chromatin distribution, and membrane contour irregularities are all more severe in HSIL than in LSIL.

Atypical squamous cells of undetermined significance (ASC-US) is a term used when the degree of non-reactive cellular abnormalities and/or number of abnormal cells does not allow a definitive diagnosis of low-grade SIL.

Atypical squamous cells, cannot exclude high-grade squamous intraepithelial lesion (ASC-H), is a term used when there is a suspicion for HSIL, but the number of cells and/or the cellular features are suggestive, but not conclusive for such a diagnosis. The cytologic pattern is usually that of small, immature cells with mild to moderate nuclear atypia (atypical squamous metaplasia), but the degree of nuclear enlargement, hyperchromasia, and membrane irregularity is insufficient for a definite diagnosis of HSIL.

Invasive squamous cell carcinoma exhibits a background of necrosis composed of amorphous granular material and erythrocytes. Smears show a population of variably pleomorphic keratinized and non-keratinized cells. The non-keratinized cells show scant cytoplasm, hyperchromatic nuclei with an irregular pattern of chromatin distribution, and visible nucleoli of variable sizes. The keratinized cells are long and spindle-shaped with small condensed nuclei (fiber cells), or they display a larger cytoplasmic body with a long "tail" (so-called tadpole cells).

Immunocytochemistry in Atypical Squamous Cells Markers can be used in ASC-US and LSIL cells to improve the diagnostic accuracy in the use of cervical cytologic specimens. Different markers can be used for single or double immunostainings. Dual biomarker technology allows for the simultaneous detection of p16 and Ki-67 positivity to provide a strong indicator of a transforming HPV infection (Fig. 3.76), i.e., a strong association with a high-grade lesion, because, under physiological conditions, the

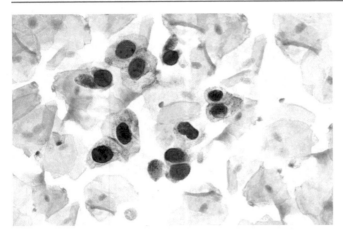

Fig. 3.76 HSIL. p16 (red) and Ki67 (brown) immunostain (high magnification)

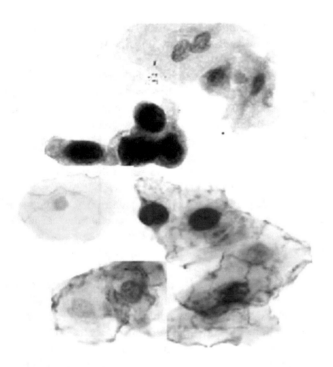

Fig. 3.77 HSIL. TOP2a (red) and MCM-2 (brown) immunostain (high magnification)

expression of one of the two markers excludes the other. Positivity for only p16 in cervical atypical cells is associated with HPV infection, but not with cellular transformation to a high-grade lesion, whereas the positivity for Ki-67 only is indicative of a reactive proliferation. Another kind of dual-biomarker immunostaining consists of a cocktail of antibodies directed against topoisomerase-2-alpha (TOP2A) and minichromosome maintenance protein-2 (MCM-2), with expression patterns similar to those for p16 and Ki67, respectively (Fig. 3.77).

Glandular Cell Abnormalities These abnormalities include endocervical and endometrial adenocarcinoma, as well as non-neoplastic conditions such as reactive/reparative and pregnancy-related changes and endocervical polyps. Depending on the severity of cellular changes present in non-neoplastic conditions, cells can be interpreted as showing "reactive endocervical cell changes," "atypical glandular cells, not otherwise specified," or they can be qualified as "favoring neoplasia" if a neoplasm is strongly favored. Reactive and reparative endocervical cells have variable degrees of nuclear enlargement, with uniform nuclei, prominent nucleoli, and slight hyperchromasia. Clinical correlation, including high-risk HPV results, and colposcopy with endocervical and endometrial curettage, are important for excluding a neoplastic process.

Endocervical adenocarcinoma in situ (AIS) consists of hyperchromatic groups of crowded cells with a characteristic "feathery" appearance, pseudostratified strips of columnar cells, and glandular formations (epithelial rosettes). Cells have large nuclei with a high nucleus-to-cytoplasm ratio, hyperchromasia with coarsely granular, evenly distributed chromatin, and sometimes small nucleoli (Fig. 3.78). Immunocytochemistry may help to differentiate between AIS and atypical reactive endocervical cells, because it is known that IMP3 immunostaining is negative in non-neoplastic endocervical cells. Furthermore, AIS cells usually show intense and widespread positivity for CEA, p16 protein, and IMP-3 (Fig. 3.79), and they have a high proliferative index tested with Ki67 antibody, whereas they are negative for bcl-2.

Invasive endocervical adenocarcinoma smears are cellular and exhibit cuboidal and columnar cells gathered in unorganized honeycomb sheets with loss of cell polarity, pseudostratified and stratified strips, papillae, and crowded hyperchromatic spherical or syncytial groups. Variable numbers of dissociated cells are also present. Cells show an increased nucleus to cytoplasm ratio, enlarged pleomorphic nuclei, coarse granular chromatin, and often macronucleoli.

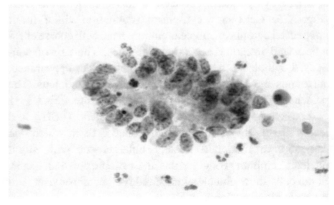

Fig. 3.78 Endocervical adenocarcinoma, Papanicolaou stain (high magnification)

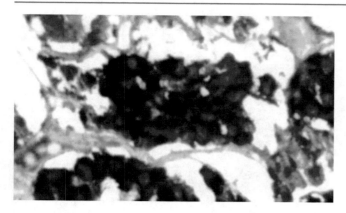

Fig. 3.79 Endocervical adenocarcinoma, IMP-3 immunostain (high magnification)

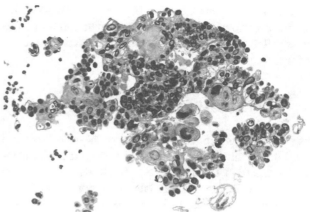

Fig. 3.80 Endometrial adenocarcinoma, H&E (high magnification)

The cytoplasm is usually thin and finely granular, or sometimes variably vacuolated, occasionally showing a signet-ring cell appearance due to mucin content.

In direct endometrial brushing, the *atypical endometrial cells* are seen isolated or in rounded clusters with scant or moderate vacuolated cytoplasm, as well as enlarged nuclei with membrane irregularity and prominent nucleoli. Similar cell changes can be seen in IUD effect, endometrial polyps, chronic endometritis, and endometrial hyperplasia.

Endometrial intraepithelial neoplasm (EIN) cells in brush cytology can appear in the form of atypical cell sheets and tubuloglandular structures. Neoplastic cells show nuclei of variable sizes, nuclear membrane irregularity, and hyperchromasia. The simultaneous positive immunostaining for Ki67 and p53 in the same cell and a negative bcl-2 immunoreaction favor the diagnosis of EIN.

Endometrial adenocarcinoma cells are cuboidal and tend to exfoliate as isolated cells and small clusters, often arranged as spheres or in very crowded three-dimensional aggregates, which are sometimes papillary (Fig. 3.80). Neoplastic cells show scant cytoplasm with blurred margins, sometimes with vacuoles of various sizes and consequent compression or peripheral displacement of the nucleus, which is mostly round with granular chromatin and irregular borders, and which contains an eosinophilic nucleolus. The well-defined nuclear membrane sometimes has peripheral granular chromatin with irregular thickening of the membrane. Rosette-like glandular features and papillary growth support the diagnosis of well-differentiated adenocarcinoma, whereas undifferentiated cells reveal their glandular origin by the characteristic eccentric positioning of the nuclei and the variably vacuolated cytoplasm. The use of immunocytochemical methods with markers such as p53 (Fig. 3.81), WT1 (Fig. 3.82), and p16 can be useful for discriminating serous

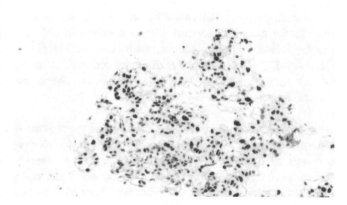

Fig. 3.81 Endometrial adenocarcinoma. p53 immunostain (high magnification)

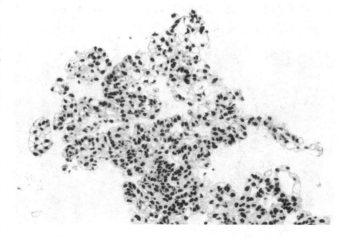

Fig. 3.82 Endometrial adenocarcinoma. WT-1 immunostain (high magnification)

endometrial carcinoma from the papillary variant of endometrioid carcinoma or benign lesions that mimic serous tumors. All three markers are positive in serous carcinoma of the endometrium.

3.11 Peritoneal Washing

This is a procedure in which isotonic saline-water solution is used for washing of the peritoneal cavity during gynecologic or digestive system surgery. Washings are collected and processed in the cytology laboratory for evaluation of the presence or absence of cancer cells in the peritoneal cavity.

Normal Peritoneal Washing The sample obtained is usually cellular and consists of mesothelial-cell sheets (forcibly exfoliated), single and clustered histiocytes, and leukocytes. Mesothelial cells show round or oval nuclei with thin and regular nuclear contours, fine chromatin, and small nucleoli. Occasionally, papillary clusters of benign mesothelial cells, as well as minute fragments of benign adipose tissue and skeletal muscle, can be observed.

Gynecologic Malignancies *Ovarian serous carcinoma* is the most common type of gynecologic cancer in which cancer cells are present in peritoneal washings. A low-grade serous carcinoma consists of small and monomorphic cells, usually organized in large tridimensional clusters, whereas single and clustered pleomorphic malignant cells characterize a high-grade tumor (Fig. 3.83). Neoplastic cells can form acinar or papillary clusters and show a vacuolated cytoplasm with mesothelium-like features. *Ovarian serous borderline tumor* (a serous tumor of low-malignant potential) exhibits a

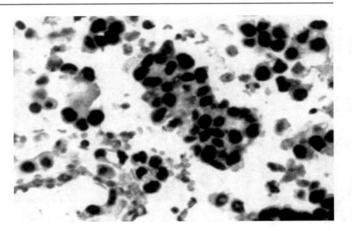

Fig. 3.84 Papillary ovary carcinoma, WT-1 immunostain (high magnification)

cytologic pattern similar to that seen in a low-grade serous carcinoma. Cells of serous borderline tumor and ovarian serous carcinoma are positive for CK7, WT-1 (Fig. 3.84), PAX-8, CA125, B72.3, and EMA. Hormonal receptor, ER, and PgR can be expressed.

Ovarian mucinous carcinoma shows single or clustered tumor cells with mucin-containing vacuolated cytoplasm and usually eccentrically placed nuclei. Neoplastic cells express CK7, B72.3, HAM56, and EMA. Some cells are also positive for CK20, PAX-8, CDX-2, CEA, MUC-2, MUC-5 AC, and WT-1. Of note, *germ-cell* and *sex-cord tumors* of the ovary rarely involve the peritoneum.

Single and clustered small cuboidal malignant epithelial cells with scant cytoplasm, enlarged monomorphic nuclei, coarse chromatin, and conspicuous nucleoli characterize the cytology of low-grade *endometrial endometrioid carcinoma* in peritoneal washings, whereas loose aggregates or clusters of variably pleomorphic neoplastic cells are seen in high-grade endometrioid carcinoma.

Papillary serous endometrial carcinoma is characterized by clustered small cuboidal cells with scant cytoplasm and enlarged hyperchromatic nuclei with inconspicuous nucleoli. A "hobnail" appearance can be observed in the cell aggregates. *Clear-cell carcinoma* contains single and clustered pleomorphic malignant cells with clear cytoplasm.

Endometrial carcinoma is positive for vimentin, CK7, CK8, CK18, CK19, ESA (Ber-Ep4), EMA, and TAG B72.3; some neoplastic cells express CK5, CK6, CK14, CK17, and PAX-8. Serous papillary and clear-cell endometrial carcinomas show intense positivity for p53, PTEN, and β-catenin. Serous papillary endometrial carcinoma cells also express WT-1 and p16.

Endocervical adenocarcinoma cells can be present in peritoneal washing, whereas squamous carcinoma cells

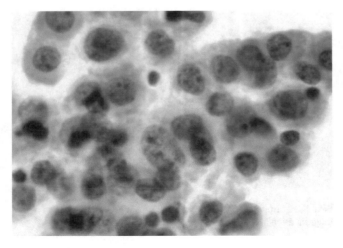

Fig. 3.83 Papillary ovary carcinoma, Papanicolaou stain (high magnification)

rarely spread. Neoplastic cells usually occur in clusters and show abundant cytoplasm, eccentric hyperchromatic nuclei, and prominent nucleoli. Neoplastic cells are positive for low-molecular-weight cytokeratins, CEA, EMA, MUC5AC, and p16. Some neoplastic cells express CDX-2.

Gastro-Enteric Carcinomas Peritoneal washing at the time of laparotomy has been used for assessment of peritoneal spreading of gastric and colonic cancer. *Gastric adenocarcinoma* cells usually appear similar to those of mucinous adenocarcinoma from other sites and usually have a signet-ring appearance. Neoplastic cells are positive for CK7 and/or CK20 or show only CK8, CK18, and CK19. HepPar antigen and pS2 protein also are helpful.

Cells derived from *adenocarcinoma of the large bowel* usually are arranged in large, compact, irregular papillary clusters of columnar glandular cells, which sometimes show a palisade or glandular arrangement. Neoplastic cells express CK20, CDX-2, CEA, and villin.

Pancreatic and Biliary Tract Carcinomas These two types of carcinomas have similar cytomorphologic characteristics. The neoplastic cells are single, but they also form sheets and irregular three-dimensional structures with nuclear crowding and overlapping. Nuclear enlargement with irregular contours, variably dense clumped chromatin, and prominent nucleoli are observed.

Neoplastic cells express low-molecular-weight cytokeratins, a DUPAN-2 marker, and various mucins. Some neoplastic cells also express CK20 and/or CK17.

Suggested Reading

Auger M, et al. A practical guide for ancillary studies in pulmonary cytologic specimens. Cancer Cytopathol. 2018;126(S8):599–614.

Botti G, et al. ProEx C as diagnostic marker for detection of urothelial carcinoma in urinary samples: a review. Int J Med Sci. 2017;14(6):554–9.

Chandra A, et al. The BSCC code of practice: exfoliative cytopathology (excluding gynecological cytopathology). Cytopathology. 2009;20:211–23.

Chawla N, et al. Role of urine cytology in bladder neoplasm: cytopathological correlation and review of literature. J Mar Med Soc. 2018;20:27–30.

Fowler LJ, Lachar WA. Application of immunohistochemistry to cytology. Arch Pathol Lab Med. 2008;132:373–83.

Idowu MO, Powers CN. Lung cancer cytology: potential pitfalls and mimics - a review. Int J Clin Exp Pathol. 2010;3(4):367–85.

Kim HJ, Yoo JH. Cytokeratin 20/p53 dual immunocytochemistry for improving the diagnostic accuracy of urine liquid-based cytology in the detection of urothelial neoplasm: a retrospective study. Cyto Journal. 2017;14:27.

Michael C. Exfoliative pulmonary cytology. In: Gattuso P, Reddy V, Masood S, editors. Differential diagnosis in cytopathology: Cambridge University Press; 2014. p. 40–86.

Norimatsu Y, et al. The role of liquid-based preparation in the evaluation of endometrial cytology. Acta Cytol. 2013;57:423–35.

Papanicolaou Society of Cytopathology Task Force on Standards of Practice. Guidelines of the papanicolaou society of cytopathology for the examination of cytologic specimens obtained from the respiratory tract. Diagn Cytopathol. 1999;21(1):61–9.

Powers CN. Diagnosis of infectious diseases: a cytopathologist's perspective. Clin Microbiol Rev. 1998;11(2):341–65.

Sun H, et al. Progress in immunocytochemical staining for cervical cancer screening. Cancer Manag Res. 2019;11:1817–27.

Zakowski MF. Cytology nomenclature and 2015 World Health Organization classification of lung cancer. Cancer Cytopathol. 2016;124(2):81–8.

Fine-needle aspiration (FNA) is a practical, minimally invasive, and minimally traumatic method used for harvesting of material for cytologic diagnosis and for performance of ancillary tests, in particular immunocytochemistry. In the great majority of cases, such a dual combination is highly sensitive and specific for the diagnosis of benign and malignant lesions, as well as of those with a high risk of neoplastic transformation, allowing the selection of patients who need to have surgery and saving patients from unnecessary surgical procedures. A palpable lesion can be approached by palpation guidance; however, it may be preferable to harvest material under ultrasound guidance; this allows the operator to visualize and select solid or non-necrotic areas of the lesion that are more likely to provide material suitable for cytologic interpretation and for performing ancillary tests, as often occurs in the cases of palpable metastatic deposits in the neck area. Ultrasound-guided FNA also allows the identification and sampling of superficial non-palpable nodules and is the preferred sampling method for lesions in the head and neck area and in the breast.

The main cytology features and helpful practical immunocytochemistry of palpable and non-palpable masses of superficial organs harvested by FNA will be covered in this chapter.

4.1 Thyroid Gland

4.1.1 Benign Thyroid Nodule

Cytologic preparations show follicular epithelial cells arranged in nicely cohesive and well-organized sheets in a background of colloid that is better visualized in Romanowsky-stained smears than in Papanicolaou-stained and liquid-based cytology smears. Occasionally, intact large thyroid follicles with a central lumen containing colloid are present. Benign follicular cells are of variable size, polygonal, and with moderate amounts of amphophilic to eosinophilic cytoplasm and show a central round nucleus with fine chromatin. Thyroid follicular cells stain with CK7, CK8, CK18, thyroglobulin, TTF-1, PAX-8, FOXE1, T3, and T4 antibodies. C cells (parafollicular) are not identifiable morphologically in normal thyroid cytologic samples; they have clear cytoplasm and oval to round nuclei and are highlighted by immunostaining with calcitonin, calcitonin gene-related peptide, chromogranin A, synaptophysin, somatostatin, and bombesin.

Macrophages can be present in cytologic preparations from benign thyroid nodules with cystic change. Variable cell degeneration is present when cystic change occurs, and cytologic preparations show follicular cells with cyst-lining metaplastic changes, atrophic features, and variable nuclear enlargement, anisonucleosis, chromatin clearing, and nuclear grooves. The macrophage nature can be proved by CD68-positive immunostaining. Hemosiderin-laden macrophages and lysed blood are seen in hemorrhagic cystic change that may be secondary to ischemia in a nodular goiter.

4.1.2 Thyroid Hyperplasia

Nodular hyperplasia Follicular cells are found to be isolated and arranged in monolayers, spheres, and intact follicles in a background of thin colloid. Follicular cells show variable amounts of cytoplasm, sometimes containing granules of lipochrome or hemosiderin. The nuclei are round to oval with inconspicuous nucleoli. There are variable amounts of Hürthle cells, macrophages, and lymphocytes. Large follicular cells may show anisonucleosis, nuclear clearing, and grooves simulating papillary thyroid carcinoma, or they may appear polygonal with large nuclei and prominent nucleoli. Immunocytochemical reactions, which are similar to those of a benign thyroid nodule, identify the normal immunophenotype of the epithelial cells.

E. Leonardo, R. H. Bardales, *Practical Immunocytochemistry in Diagnostic Cytology*,
https://doi.org/10.1007/978-3-030-46656-5_4

Graves' disease (toxic diffuse hyperplasia) This is an autoimmune disease that is caused by the development of autoantibodies directed against thyroid antigens such as thyroglobulin, thyroid peroxidase, and the thyroid-stimulating hormone (TSH) receptor. These autoantibodies can either stimulate or inhibit thyroid function. The stimulation of TSH receptors promotes the production of thyroid hormones that causes hyperthyroidism. Microscopically, the cytologic preparations are usually cellular, composed of cohesive cuboidal or columnar cells with abundant slightly clear cytoplasm, a round nucleus, and conspicuous nucleoli. Small aggregates of follicular cells, lymphocytes, and Hürthle cells may be present. Thyroid follicular and Hürthle cells show their normal immunophenotype. Infiltrating lymphocytes are mainly T cells that are CD4-positive and partly also express CD25, whereas B cells, which are positive for CD19 and CD20, are rare. Occasionally, lymphocytes may express aberrant IGF receptors.

Smears from colloid-rich hyperplastic nodules show abundant colloid, large numbers of follicular cells, and immunostains that are like those of normal follicular cells.

4.1.3 Thyroiditis

Acute thyroiditis The cytologic samples show necrotic debris, numerous granulocytes and histiocytes, and scant follicular epithelium, often with reparative/regenerative changes. Follicular cells have the immunophenotype of normal follicular thyroid cells.

Chronic (lymphocytic) thyroiditis The cytology is characterized by a mixture of follicular and inflammatory cells. The follicular cells form small, two-dimensional, cohesive clusters and have densely granular oncocytic cytoplasm. They have enlarged, sometimes grooved nuclei with a variable presence of nucleoli. Two different populations of Hürthle cells are recognized. The first type (identifiable by an intensely eosinophilic and granular cytoplasm) delimits the small thyroid follicles and variably stains with anti-thyroglobulin antibodies. The second type appears to be less eosinophilic, is found less frequently, and has no thyroglobulin immunoreactivity, whereas it is positive for somatostatin and for NSE. Occasionally, the follicular cells display marked atypia and nuclear grooves. Sometimes "flame" cells, squamous metaplastic cells, and giant cells are observed. There is an intense inflammatory infiltrate composed of lymphocytes, sometimes grouped with formation of lymphoid follicles, histiocytes, and plasma cells. Lymphocytes are composed of prevalent T cells, which show positivity for CD2, CD3, CD4, CD5, CD7, and CD8, and

rare B-lymphocytes positive for CD19, CD20, CD79a, and PAX-5. Some lymphocytes are immunostained with CD10 and bcl-6, demonstrating their origin from germinal centers. B cells and plasma cells are not light-chain-restricted.

Subacute thyroiditis (De Quervain's thyroiditis) Cytologic samples are usually hypocellular and consist of granulomas composed of epithelioid histiocytes, multinucleated giant cells, and variable amounts of dense and granular colloid. Variable numbers of lymphocytes, plasma cells, eosinophils, and neutrophils are sometimes present. Follicular thyroid cells are generally sparse and can show degenerative together with reactive changes.

CD68 and CD163 immunostainings allow identification of the histiocytic nature of epithelioid cells, whereas anti-thyroglobulin and TTF-1 are positive in follicular cells. Rare cells have immunostaining positivity for somatostatin.

Riedel's thyroiditis (also known as fibrous thyroiditis, sclerosing thyroiditis, or Riedel's ligneous struma) Cytologic aspirates are often unsatisfactory for diagnosis due to sparse cellularity. Cytologic samples show fragments of fibrous tissue and few inflammatory cells, whereas follicular thyroid epithelium is usually absent. Immunocytochemical stains of the follicular cells that are present are like the normal follicular cells. Plasma cells usually show IgG4 positivity. The main clinical differential diagnosis is the sclerosing type of anaplastic carcinoma; the two entities have a similar clinical presentation, including anterior lower neck, esophageal, and airway compressive symptoms.

4.1.4 Follicular Neoplasms

Adenomas This group of follicular lesions of the thyroid includes non-papillary follicular patterned lesions (follicular adenoma and follicular carcinoma) and Hürthle cell neoplasms (oncocytic adenoma and oncocytic carcinoma). The diagnostic criteria for differentiating adenoma from carcinoma are based not on cellular characteristics, but on histologic features, such as capsular and lymphovascular invasion or the presence of distant metastases. Because it is not possible to distinguish between adenoma and carcinoma on cytologic FNA preparations, surgical excision of the nodule is necessary for a definitive diagnosis. Microscopically, the cytologic FNA usually has high cellularity, with a paucity of colloid. The follicular cells are bland-appearing and are arranged in three-dimensional clusters as well as microfollicular or trabecular arrangements (Fig. 4.1). Follicular cells are usually larger than normal and usually do not show nuclear atypia, pleomorphism, or mitoses. Hürthle cell neoplasms are similar to follicular adenomas, but are made up of oncocytic cells (Fig. 4.2).

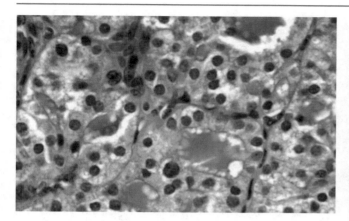

Fig. 4.1 Follicular adenoma. H&E (high magnification)

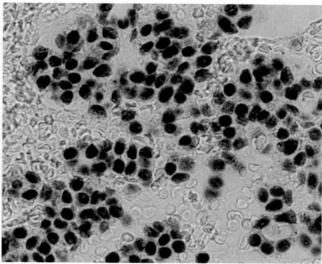

Fig. 4.3 Follicular adenoma. TTF-1 immunostain (high magnification)

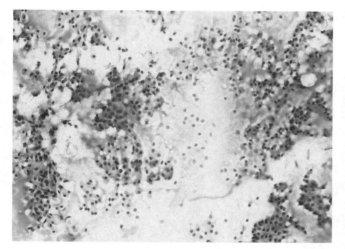

Fig. 4.2 Oncocytic adenoma. H&E (high magnification)

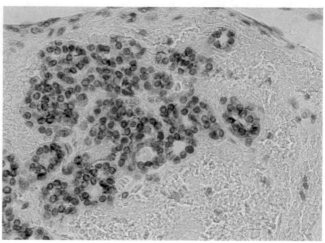

Fig. 4.4 Follicular adenoma. CD56 immunostain (high magnification)

The cells of follicular cell adenoma show positivity for TTF-1 (Fig. 4.3), CD56 (Fig. 4.4), thyroglobulin (Fig. 4.5), CK7, CK8, CK18, EMA, CD44v, and COX-2, whereas they are negative for CK19 (Fig. 4.6), HBME-1 (Fig. 4.7), and galectin-3 (Fig. 4.8). Some cells may express RET. Oncocytic adenomas (Fig. 4.9), as well as the cells of follicular and Hürthle cell carcinomas, exhibit a similar immunophenotype: positivity for CK7, CK8, CK18, TTF-1, thyroperoxidase, thyroglobulin, EMA, CD44v6, CD56 (Fig. 4.10), and COX-2. HBME-1 (Fig. 4.11), galectin-3 (Fig. 4.12), CK19 (Fig. 4.13), and RET are usually negative or expressed only in few cells.

4.1.5 Hyalinizing Trabecular Tumor

The cytologic FNA preparations show variable cellularity, consisting of scattered cells, monolayers, and small groups of cohesive follicular cells. Characteristic branching papillary fragments supported by fibrillary stroma instead of a

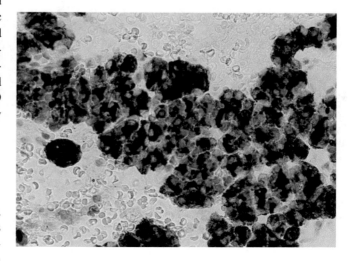

Fig. 4.5 Follicular adenoma. Thyroglobulin immunostain (high magnification)

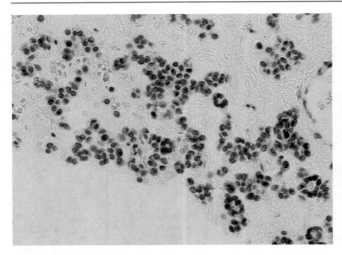

Fig. 4.6 Follicular adenoma. CK19 immunostain (high magnification)

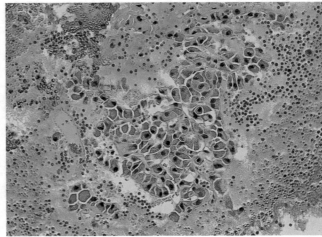

Fig. 4.9 Oncocytic adenoma. H&E (high magnification)

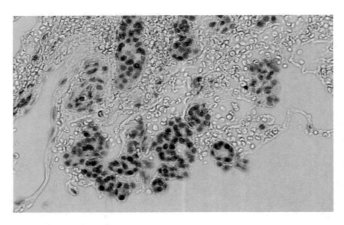

Fig. 4.7 Follicular adenoma. HBME-1 immunostain (high magnification)

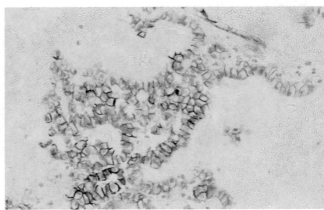

Fig. 4.10 Oncocytic adenoma. CD56 immunostain (high magnification)

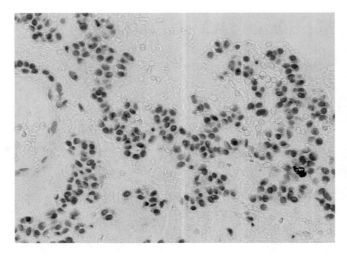

Fig. 4.8 Follicular adenoma. Galectin-3 immunostain (high magnification)

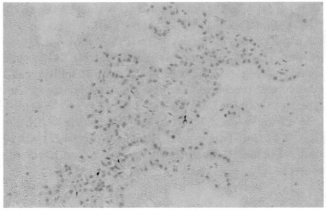

Fig. 4.11 Oncocytic adenoma. HBME-1 immunostain (high magnification)

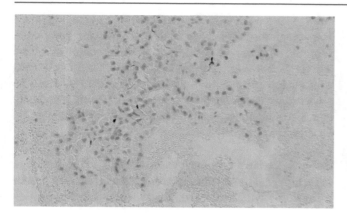

Fig. 4.12 Oncocytic adenoma. Galectin-3 immunostain (high magnification)

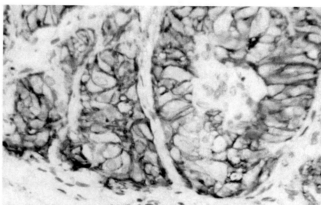

Fig. 4.15 Hyalinizing trabecular tumor. MIB-1 immunostain (high magnification)

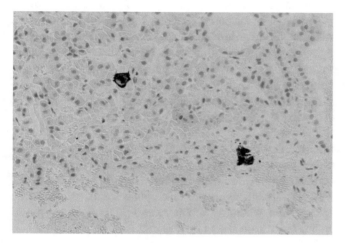

Fig. 4.13 Oncocytic adenoma. CK19 immunostain (high magnification)

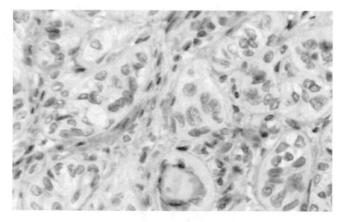

Fig. 4.14 Hyalinizing trabecular tumor. Romanowsky stain (high magnification)

fibrovascular core are often seen. Sometimes, a trabecular pattern with "palisade" cells can be observed (Fig. 4.14). The epithelial cells are round to oval with abundant filamentous, vacuolated, and ill-defined eosinophilic cytoplasm. Nuclei

are mildly pleomorphic, located eccentrically, with fine dispersed chromatin and occasional small nucleoli. Nuclear pseudoinclusions are usually numerous, and grooves can be observed. Tumor cells are positive for thyroglobulin, CD56, TTF-1, PAX-8, and collagen IV. Some cells express galectin-3. A characteristic is the membranous and cytoplasmic MIB-1 staining pattern (Fig. 4.15).

4.1.6 Papillary Thyroid Carcinoma (PTC)

Classical variant In cytological preparations, PTC may show papillary structures with fibrovascular cores, which are a diagnostic criterion. In other cases, the papillary formations are missing, and the neoplastic cells are arranged in crowded layers. The diagnosis of PTC is based on the nuclear characteristics along with the architecture of the tissue fragments and psammoma bodies when these are present. The neoplastic cells have a variable cytoplasm, which can be scarce or abundant, vacuolated, or the dense metaplastic type or oncocytic (Figs. 4.16 and 4.17). The nuclei are enlarged and crowded, with pale, powdery chromatin, longitudinal grooves, and sharply defined nuclear pseudoinclusions. The neoplastic cells usually have a nucleolus of variable size, usually small. Colloid is usually present and sometimes abundant, with anomalous viscosity (so-called "bubble gum-type" colloid). Psammomatous calcifications may also be present.

Follicular variant Smears show follicular cells that are arranged in small- or medium-sized follicles showing nuclear grooves, occasional nuclear pseudoinclusions, and dense, thick colloid in the follicular lumen. The cytologic pattern is similar, if not identical, to that seen in noninvasive follicular thyroid neoplasm with papillary-like nuclear features (NIFTP), an indolent tumor that is only diagnosed histologically.

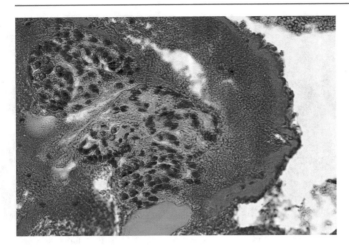

Fig. 4.16 Papillary thyroid carcinoma. H&E (high magnification)

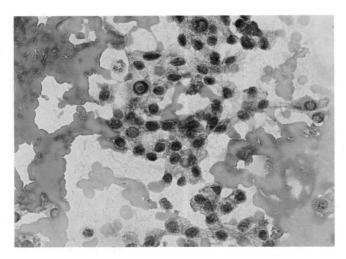

Fig. 4.17 Papillary thyroid carcinoma. Papanicolaou stain (high magnification)

Diffuse sclerosing variant Cell preparations have poor cellularity, with the presence of psammoma bodies and a background of chronic inflammation. Neoplastic cells show the typical nuclear features of PTC and occasionally those of squamous metaplasia.

Cystic variant FNA often yields poor epithelial cellularity and is often diagnosed as inadequate for cytologic interpretation. There is an inflammatory background, debris, and numerous macrophages with variable cytoplasmic hemosiderin that may obscure the neoplastic cells often arranged in small aggregates, papillae, and small follicles. Although the cellularity is low, it is usually sufficient to allow one to recognize the nuclear features of PTC. Cyst-lining cells with reactive/regenerative or metaplastic-type features can be observed.

Oncocytic variant The cytologic samples show a pure population of usually large oncocytic cells which are isolated or

arranged in sheets, as well as papillae or syncytial fragments. The neoplastic cells have abundant granular cytoplasm, eccentric nuclei with dense and granular chromatin, and prominent nucleoli. A variable number of neoplastic cells with nuclear grooves and nuclear pseudoinclusions can be observed. In the presence of a prominent papillary architecture and numerous lymphoid cells, a *Warthin-like variant* must be considered.

Tall-cell variant Cytology shows papillary fragments of large, polygonal, and tall neoplastic cells with abundant dense eosinophilic cytoplasm and nuclei with pseudoinclusions.

Columnar-cell variant Cytologic samples show neoplastic cells arranged in aggregates, sheets, and syncytial tissue fragments that show a papillary configuration, sometimes with fibrovascular cores. Cells have a monomorphic aspect with a palisade arrangement, and they show a pale and clear cytoplasm, pseudostratified nuclei with finely granular chromatin, and small or inconspicuous nucleoli. The cytologic pattern resembles that seen in cell aggregates of endometrial origin. Few or no neoplastic cells with nuclear features of PTC may be identified.

Cribriform-morular variant Cytologic samples show elongated cancer cells arranged in papillary, cribriform, and morular aggregates with characteristic nuclear features of PTC. A variable number of macrophages may be seen in the background, whereas "bubble gum-type" colloid and psammoma bodies are absent or very rare.

The neoplastic cells of the classic histotype of papillary thyroid carcinoma and most of its variants are positive for thyroglobulin (Fig. 4.18), TTF-1 (Fig. 4.19), HBME-1 (Fig. 4.20), CK19 (Fig. 4.21), galectin-3 (Fig. 4.22), COX-2, and TROP-2. Variable numbers of neoplastic cells are also positive for

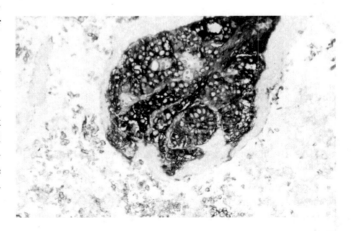

Fig. 4.18 Papillary thyroid carcinoma. Thyroglobulin immunostain (high magnification)

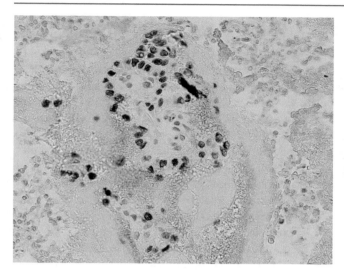

Fig. 4.19 Papillary thyroid carcinoma. TTF-1 immunostain (high magnification)

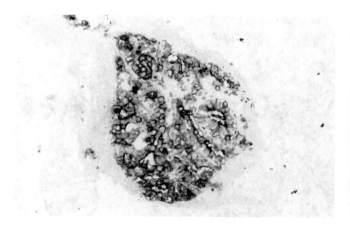

Fig. 4.20 Papillary thyroid carcinoma. HBME-1 immunostain (high magnification)

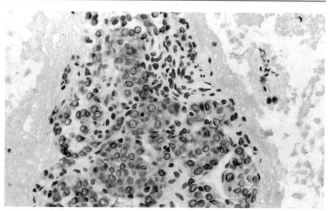

Fig. 4.21 Papillary thyroid carcinoma. CK19 immunostain (high magnification)

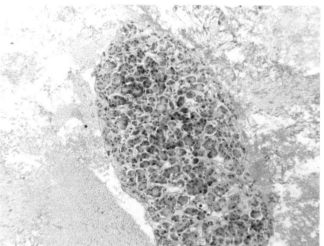

Fig. 4.22 Papillary thyroid carcinoma. Galectin-3 immunostain (high magnification)

CD15 and p63 and for some carbohydrate antigens, such as CA19.9. In contrast, in the cribriform-morular variant of PTC, the neoplastic cells are negative for thyroglobulin and TTF-1. In the morules, CK19 is expressed weakly, whereas there is strong positivity for CD10, E-cadherin, and bcl-2.

4.1.7 Poorly Differentiated (Insular) Carcinoma

FNA shows high cellularity in a nesting (insular) and trabecular pattern, including crowded groups of follicular cells and some microfollicles in a background of very little or absent colloid. Single cells can also be seen, sometimes with a plasmacytoid appearance. Neoplastic cells lack features of PTC and are small and monomorphic, with scant, delicate cytoplasm, small round or convoluted hyperchromatic nuclei, and inconspicuous nucleoli. Background necrosis and mitoses are frequently identified.

Neoplastic cells are positive for thyroglobulin, with the characteristic paranuclear immunostaining pattern that appears as a globule (dot-like) in the Golgian area or is shaped like a nuclear "hood." CK7, CK8, CK18, CK19, TTF-1, thyroperoxidase (TPO), EMA, PAX-8, T3, and T4 are also expressed. Groups of neoplastic elements can also express vimentin, TPO, CA 19.9, CA 50, HBME-1, galectin-3, CD44v6, and bcl-2. Neoplastic cells can have BRAF, p53, and β-catenin expression on immunocytochemistry.

4.1.8 Undifferentiated (Anaplastic) Carcinoma

Cytologic specimens show necrosis, high cellularity, and highly pleomorphic, often discohesive malignant cells. A dispersed single-cell pattern is common, sometimes with numerous naked nuclei found in the background. Neoplastic cells have moderate to abundant cytoplasm, highly pleomorphic enlarged nuclei with irregular nuclear membranes, dark, irregular chromatin clumping, macronucleoli, and occasional intranuclear pseudoinclusions (Fig. 4.23). Atypical mitoses may be seen. Cancer cells may have squamoid features, have a spindle appearance, or be giant-multinucleated (osteoclast-like) or there may be a combination of these cell types.

Immunocytochemistry shows positivity for CK7 (Fig. 4.24), CK8, CK18, CK19, PAX-8, p53, and vimentin. Thyroglobulin, TTF-1, thyroperoxidase, galectin-3, CEA, EMA, T3, and T4 are usually negative or expressed in rare neoplastic cells.

4.1.9   Medullary Thyroid Carcinoma (MTC)

FNA samples show moderate to high cellularity in aggregates and single neoplastic cells with mild to moderate pleomorphism (Fig. 4.25). MTC cells may appear small, round, cuboidal, spindle, plasmacytoid, oncocytic, pigmented, squamoid, clear, giant, and/or pleomorphic, arranged in a tubular, papillary, lobular, islet, or solid growth. Neuroendocrine features including cytoplasmic granules, round and eccentric nuclei with "salt-and-pepper" chromatin, and inconspicuous nucleoli can be observed (Fig. 4.26). In most cases, amorphous material related to amyloid is present in the background. Psammoma bodies may occasionally be present.

The immunocytochemical pattern is characterized by positivity for CK7 (Fig. 4.27), CK8, CK18, CK19, calcitonin (Fig. 4.28), chromogranin A (Fig. 4.29), synaptophysin (Fig. 4.30), CEA (Fig. 4.31), PAX-8 (Fig. 4.32), p53, and vimentin. Thyroglobulin (Fig. 4.33), TTF-1, thyroperoxidase, galectin-3, CEA, EMA, T3, and T4 are usually negative or expressed in rare neoplastic cells.

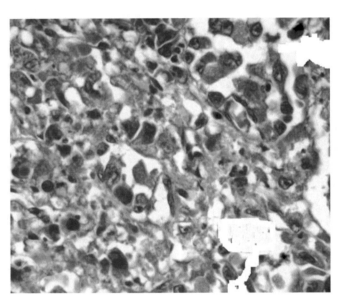

Fig. 4.23 Anaplastic carcinoma H&E (high magnification)

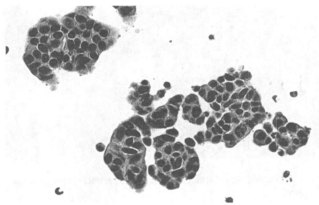

Fig. 4.25 Medullary carcinoma. H&E (high magnification)

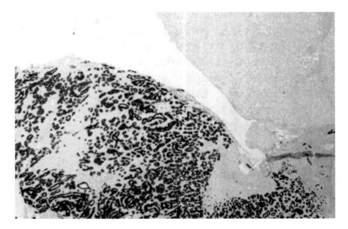

Fig. 4.24 Anaplastic carcinoma. CK7 immunostain (high magnification)

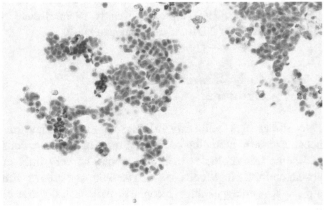

Fig. 4.26 Medullary carcinoma. Romanowsky stain (high magnification)

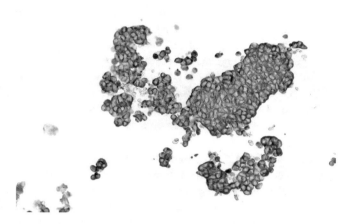

Fig. 4.27 Medullary carcinoma. CK7 immunostain (high magnification)

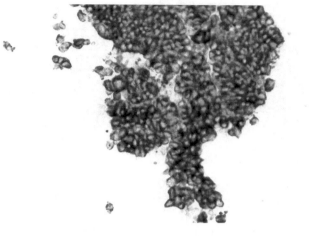

Fig. 4.30 Medullary carcinoma. Synaptophysin immunostain (high magnification)

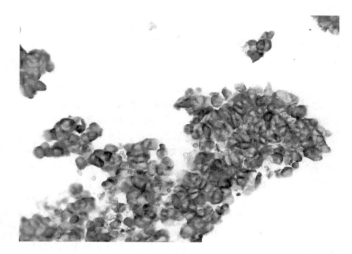

Fig. 4.28 Medullary carcinoma. Calcitonin immunostain (high magnification)

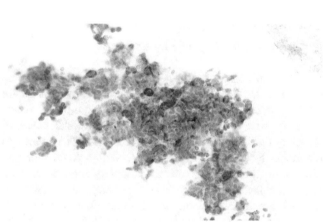

Fig. 4.31 Medullary carcinoma. CEA immunostain (high magnification)

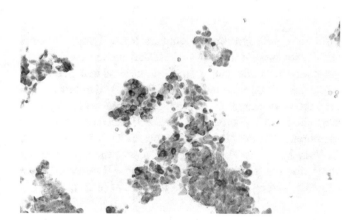

Fig. 4.29 Medullary carcinoma. Chromogranin A immunostain (high magnification)

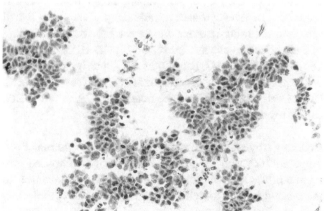

Fig. 4.32 Medullary carcinoma. PAX-8 immunostain (high magnification)

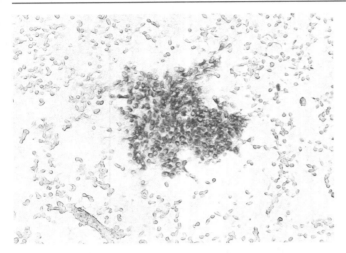

Fig. 4.33 Medullary carcinoma. Thyroglobulin immunostain (high magnification)

4.1.10 Primary Thyroid Lymphoma

All of the different histotypes of primary lymphoma can be observed in the thyroid gland; however, the most frequent are diffuse large B-cell, mucosa-associated lymphoid tissue (MALT), and follicular lymphomas. Occasional cases of T-cell lymphoma have been reported. The FNA cytologic diagnosis, by experienced observers, is often positive or suspicious for lymphoma. However, ancillary procedures such as immunocytochemistry, flow cytometry, and molecular biology are necessary for an accurate diagnosis and for proper classification of the lymphoproliferative process. The screening panel of antibodies commonly used in flow cytometry includes CD3, CD4, CD5, CD8, CD10, CD19, CD20, CD30, CD45, CD56, and lambda and kappa light chains. If the results of flow cytometry guide the presence of a B-cell lymphoma, further markers can be used for better definition of the diagnosis, such as CD11c, CD22, CD23, CD25, CD43, CD103, CD200, bcl-2, bcl-6, IgM, IgG, and IgA. In the case of T-cell lymphoma, additional markers, such as CD1a, CD2, CD7, CD16, CD57, TCR alpha/beta, and TCR gamma/delta, can be used.

Primary thyroid diffuse large B-cell lymphoma FNA preparation cytology shows high cellularity, composed predominantly with a monomorphic population of medium- to large-sized lymphoid cells with a high nuclear/cytoplasmic ratio and scant cytoplasm. There are round to oval nuclei, fine chromatin, a central nucleolus, or 1–3 eccentrically located nucleoli; some cells show irregular nuclear contours. Few small lymphocytes, macrophages, plasma cells, and occasional thyroid follicular cells can be observed. Immunostains identify two main immunophenotypic features of large B-cell lymphomas: one consistent with the fol-

licular center origin (GCB subtype) and the other compatible with large activated B cells (ABC subtype). Both subtypes express strong surface CD20, CD79a, and PAX-5. The GCB subtype may be diagnosed if there is expression of CD10 and/or bcl-6 and a lack of MUM1. Alternatively, the lack of CD10, but presence of bcl-6 without MUM1, also points to GCB. The ABC subtype must be MUM1-positive and CD10-negative, whereas bcl-6 expression may be present.

In cases of MALT lymphoma, the FNA cytology reveals a heterogeneous population of lymphoid cells consisting of small- and intermediate-sized lymphocytes with scant pale cytoplasm, round to irregular sometimes indented nuclei, finely granular chromatin, and small central nucleoli. Plasmacytoid, lymphoplasmacytic, and monocytoid cells can be present.

Immunocytochemistry or flow cytometry is essential for distinguishing lymphoma from lymphocytic thyroiditis.

MALT-type lymphoma FNA smears show a heterogeneous population of small- and intermediate-sized lymphocytes with scant pale cytoplasm, irregular nuclei, finely granular chromatin, and small central nucleoli. Plasmacytoid, lymphoplasmacytic, and monocytoid cells can be present. Immunocytochemistry or flow cytometry is essential for distinguishing lymphoma from lymphocytic thyroiditis. This lymphoma pattern shows positive staining for CD19, CD20, CD79a, and PAX-5. Sometimes, there is co-expression of CD43, whereas CD3, CD5, and CD10 are negative. Flow cytometry shows the presence of monoclonality of light-chain immunoglobulins. However, it is necessary to interpret this result with caution, as there are clusters of lymphocytes infiltrating in lymphocytic thyroiditis that may be clonal. Molecular biology shows a t(11;18) translocation.

Follicular cell lymphoma Smears show lymphoid cells with scant cytoplasm and an indented nucleus with finely granular chromatin and a small or non-evident nucleolus, which are mixed with larger lymphoid cells that have abundant pale cytoplasm, as well as large nuclei with dispersed chromatin and 1–3 prominent nucleoli placed on the nuclear membrane. The neoplastic cells express CD10, CD19, CD20, CD79a, bcl-2, bcl-6, PAX-5, and clonal membrane light-chain immunoglobulins. Most follicular lymphomas are characterized by the translocation t(14; 18) (q32; q21).

Primary T-cell lymphoma This type of lymphoma of the thyroid gland is extremely rare; very few cases have been reported in the literature. Most T-cell lymphomas are associated with Hashimoto's thyroiditis; it is difficult to assess their neoplastic nature, even with the use of immunocytochemistry. However, neoplastic T-lymphocytes show T-cell-restricted markers such as CD2, CD3, CD4, and/or CD8,

CD5, and CD7. Rearrangement of T-cell receptor is necessary for confirming the diagnosis.

4.1.11 Metastases to the Thyroid

Although rare, non-primary thyroid malignancies are caused mainly by direct spread of primary carcinomas of the pharynx, larynx, and the upper third of the esophagus. However, the thyroid gland can be involved by metastasis from kidney, colorectum, stomach, lung, and breast carcinomas, melanoma, as well as sarcomas, leukemias, and lymphomas. FNA specimens are usually cellular and are composed of neoplastic cells mixed with normal follicular thyroid cells. Usually, the cytologic aspect of metastatic cells is similar to that of the primary tumor, but in most cases, poorly differentiated or anaplastic primary thyroid cancer must be excluded.

Metastatic clear-cell renal cell carcinoma (Fig. 4.34) Cytology may mimic a primary thyroid follicular neoplasm with predominance of macrophages. CD10 (Fig. 4.35) and renal cell carcinoma-associated marker (RCC) (Fig. 4.36) positivity allows identifying the renal origin of the neoplastic cells. Metastatic cells of the papillary renal carcinoma and papillary variant of clear-cell renal carcinoma may show nuclear indentations, grooves, and inclusions simulating a PTC. Metastatic renal cells are positive for AMACR and/or CD10 and negative for TTF-1. The oncocytic feature of the chromophobe renal cell metastases can be confused with cells of Hürthle adenoma/carcinoma. Thyroid follicular cells show TTF-1 positivity, whereas renal cells are positive for CD117.

Metastatic breast cancer Breast cancer cells can exhibit variable morphology; they can simulate medullary carcinoma, PTC, and anaplastic thyroid carcinoma. The breast

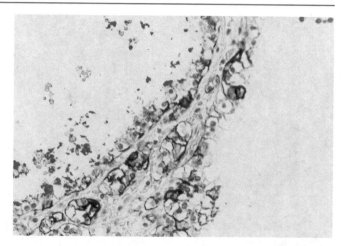

Fig. 4.35 Metastasis of clear-cell renal cell carcinoma. CD10 immunostain (high magnification)

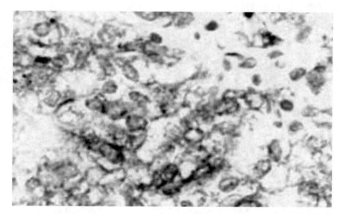

Fig. 4.36 Metastasis of clear-cell renal cell carcinoma. RCC immunostain (high magnification)

origin of the neoplastic cells can be recognized by mammaglobin and GATA-3 positivity.

Metastatic lung carcinoma The cell pattern can mimic undifferentiated cells of thyroid carcinoma: TTF-1-positive and PAX-8-negative cells are suggestive of lung cancer metastatic origin.

Metastatic colorectal adenocarcinoma Neoplastic columnar cells (Fig. 4.37) can imitate the columnar cell variant of PTC. Immunocytochemistry for CK7 and CK20 is useful for differentiating tumors of thyroid follicular origin (CK7-positive) from intestinal metastatic cells, which are positive for CK20 (Fig. 4.38) and CDX-2 (Fig. 4.39) and negative for CK7 (Fig. 4.40).

Metastatic amelanotic melanoma Melanoma cells with their polymorphism and pleomorphism can mimic medullary thyroid carcinoma cells. The positive immunos-

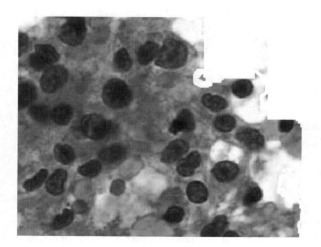

Fig. 4.34 Metastasis of clear-cell renal cell carcinoma. H&E (high magnification)

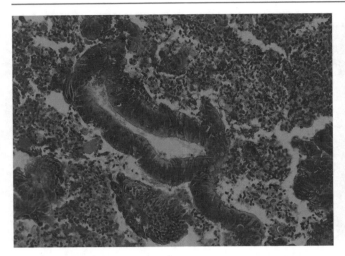

Fig. 4.37 Metastasis of colon carcinoma. H&E (high magnification)

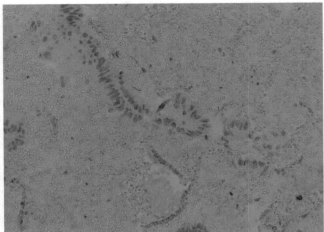

Fig. 4.40 Metastasis of colon carcinoma. CK7 immunostain (high magnification)

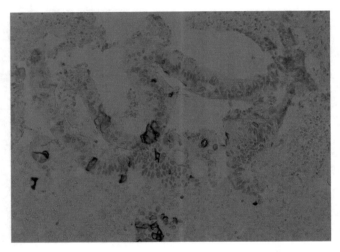

Fig. 4.38 Metastasis of colon carcinoma. CK20 immunostain (high magnification)

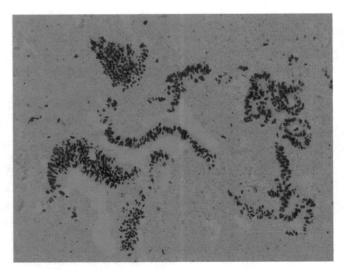

Fig. 4.39 Metastasis of colon carcinoma. CDX-2 immunostain (high magnification)

taining for melan A and HMB-45 allows identifying the cells of the melanoma.

4.2   Parathyroid Gland

4.2.1   Parathyroid Tumors

Parathyroid carcinoma, adenoma, and hyperplastic lesions have a similar cytomorphology in FNA cytology and cannot be differentiated from each other. FNA specimens of enlarged parathyroid glands are cellular and can show dispersed single cells, cohesive sheets, ribbon-like cords, complex aggregates, microfollicles, and pseudopapillary architecture. The cellularity is made up mainly of chief cells: round or cuboidal cells with scant cytoplasm, round or oval eccentric nuclei with granular coarse chromatin, and inconspicuous nucleoli (Fig. 4.41). Variable quantities of cells with large, clear vacuolated cytoplasm, a peripherally located nucleus, and cells with eosinophilic granular cytoplasm (oxyphilic cells) can be observed.

Immunocytochemical stains show the same immunophenotypic profile in both adenomas and carcinomas: positivity for CK8, CK18, CK19, chromogranin A, synaptophysin, neurofilaments, and parathormone (PTH) (Fig. 4.42). Some cells can be positive for CK7, CK14, GLUT-4, bcl-2, gp200, and vimentin.

On FNA, a parathyroid adenoma can be confused with a follicular thyroid lesion (adenoma/carcinoma). TTF-1- or PTH-positive cells identify the origin of the lesion.

If clear parathyroid cells predominate in the cytologic sample, a differential diagnosis should be made between a parathyroid adenoma and the metastasis of a clear-cell renal cell carcinoma. A PTH-positive immunoreaction and renal marker negativity allow one to make the correct diagnosis.

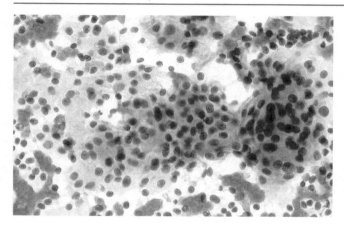

Fig. 4.41 Parathyroid carcinoma. Papanicolaou stain (high magnification)

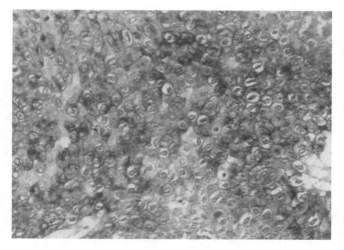

Fig. 4.42 Parathyroid carcinoma. Paratohormone immunostain (high magnification)

FNA of parathyroid lesions with a prominent oxyphilic component can be mistaken for thyroid lesions with onco-cytic features such as Hashimoto's thyroiditis, Hürthle cell neoplasms, as well as oxyphilic PTC and medullary thyroid carcinoma. Diagnostic problems can be resolved by use of a selective panel of immunocytochemical stains including PTH, thyroglobulin, TTF-1, and calcitonin. When pleomorphic cells of parathyroid adenoma predominate, the cytologic sample can mimic extra-adrenal paraganglioma (carotid body tumor): PTH-immunopositive cells of parathyroid adenoma are seen.

4.3 Salivary Gland

4.3.1 Normal Salivary Gland

FNA samples of normal salivary gland show variable cellularity composed of predominantly acinar cells, occasional ductal cells, and rare myoepithelial cells, stromal elements, and lymphocytes. Acinar cells are arranged in small, round, cohesive grape-like clusters. Two different types of acinar cells can be observed: serous and mucinous. The serous-type acinar cells are large, pyramidal, with foamy, basophilic, and granular cytoplasm and small, eccentric, round to oval nuclei with non-apparent nucleoli. The mucinous-type acinar cells are columnar, with pale cytoplasm and flattened basal nuclei. The predominance of either of the two cell types varies in the salivary glands: serous cells in the parotid and mainly mucinous cells in the minor salivary glands, while in the submandibular glands, a mixture of the two cell types is observed. The fragility of the cytoplasm of acinar cells often leads to the rupture of cells during cytological preparations and the presence of naked nuclei. Depending on their type, ductal cells can have various shapes: a low cuboidal with very scant, dense cytoplasm (intercalated ductal cells), a columnar with abundant eosinophilic cytoplasm (striated ductal cells), and a columnar with a squamous appearance (excretory ductal cells).

Acinar cells express CK7, CK8, CK18, and CK19, whereas ductal cells are positive for CK8, CK14, CK17, CK18, CK19, and EMA. Myoepithelial cells, if present, can be identified by immunostaining with CK5, CK14, CK15, CK17, α-SMA, calponin, and S-100 protein.

4.3.2 Inflammatory and Infectious Lesions

Acute and chronic sialadenitis as well as lymphoepithelial and granulomatous lesions will be covered in this section.

Acute sialadenitis FNA specimens show small clusters of acinar and ductal cells mixed with fibrin, necrotic cells, cellular debris, numerous neutrophils, varying numbers of lymphocytes, and histiocytes/macrophages. A part of the cytologic aspirate should be used for microbiological investigations.

Chronic sialadenitis The cytologic pattern is characterized by the presence of sparse acinar cells, small clusters of basaloid ductal cells, proteinaceous debris, lymphocytes, and histiocytes. Sometimes, squamous and mucinous metaplastic cells and extracellular mucin can be present.

The *sclerosing form (Küttner tumor)* is a particular type of chronic sialadenitis in which, in addition to the cytologic aspects of the classical form, a discrete quantity of plasma cells and a variable number of fibroblasts and sclerotic tissue fragments are present. Currently, it is considered to be part of the spectrum of IgG-4 disease.

Immunocytochemical staining in chronic and acute sialadenitis is unnecessary except in the sclerosing form, in which the IgG4-positive plasma cells allow the diagnosis of a Küttner tumor.

Lymphoepithelial sialadenitis (LESA) Cytologic samples are highly cellular and are composed of single and aggregated small mature lymphocytes, scattered intermediate-sized and larger lymphocytes, plasma cells, and germinal center cells. Lymphoepithelial complexes composed of polygonal and spindle ductal cells admixed with lymphoid elements and deposits of eosinophilic hyaline matter can be observed. Acinar cells are usually absent. Epithelial cells express the cytokeratins of ductal elements, whereas myoepithelial specific markers are negative. The lymphocyte population is composed mainly of T-lymphocytes, which are recognizable by immunostaining for CD2, CD3, CD5, and CD7, with a CD4/CD8 normal ratio. Some lymphocytes express markers of the B-cell line, such as CD20, CD79a, and PAX-5, and some cells are positive for the germinal center markers CD10 and bcl-6. However, it is also important to use flow cytometry to rule out the presence of a MALT-like lymphoma, because the presence of monoclonal B-lymphocytes often cannot be diagnosed by use of immunocytochemistry.

Granulomatous sialadenitis It can be associated with infections, sarcoidosis, and sometimes neoplasia. FNA specimens are characterized by aggregates of epithelioid histiocytes, which are frequently multinucleated, admixed with a background of inflammatory cells and granular necrotic cell debris all present in variable proportions. Caseous necrosis is only suggestive, but not specific for tuberculosis. Microbiological investigation, special stains, and molecular biology are necessary for making the correct diagnosis.

4.3.3 Benign Salivary Gland Tumors

Most neoplasms of the salivary glands are benign, slow-growing, and generally solitary. The parotid is the most commonly involved gland, followed by the submandibular gland. Benign tumors include pleomorphic adenoma (mixed tumor), Warthin tumor (formerly known as papillary cystadenoma lymphomatosum), oncocytoma, basal cell adenoma, canalicular adenoma, sebaceous adenoma, myoepithelioma, and intraductal papilloma.

Pleomorphic adenoma (PA) is the most frequent salivary gland tumor. FNA samples obtained from PA have a gelatinous consistency and are composed of ductal cells, myoepithelial cells, and a mesenchymal substance (Fig. 4.43). Ductal cells can be dispersed or gathered in aggregates forming sheets, tubular structures, or acini. These cells are usually small or cuboidal and show round, regular nuclei with fine chromatin and inconspicuous nucleoli. Sometimes, the epithelial cells may show squamous, mucinous, oncocytic, or sebaceous metaplasia. The myoepithelial cells are generally dispersed or aggregated in small groups and have a fusiform

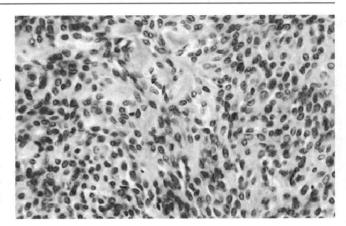

Fig. 4.43 Salivary gland pleomorphic adenoma. H&E stain (high magnification)

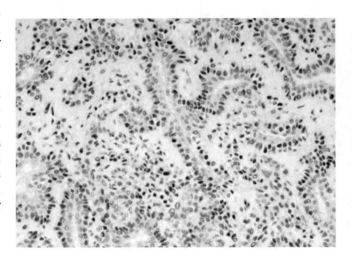

Fig. 4.44 Salivary gland pleomorphic adenoma. PLAG-1 immunostain (high magnification)

or plasmacytic-like appearance. The mesenchymal substance appears as a red to dark purple (metachromatic) fibrillary and chondromyxoid material when the cytological preparation is May–Grünwald–Giemsa-stained, whereas in Papanicolaou stain the mesenchymal substance appears pale pink to gray. The myoepithelial elements show the characteristic immunoreactivity for CK5, CK6, CK14, CK17, p63, α-SMA, calponin, smooth muscle myosin, PLAG-1 (Fig. 4.44), and S-100 protein. Myoepithelial spindle cells can also express vimentin and BMP (bone morphogenetic protein).

The ductal portion is positive for CK7, CK8, CK18, CK19, EMA, CEA, lysozyme, α-1-antitrypsin, α-1-antichimotrypsin, and lactoferrin. Some of these cells may also have immunopositivity for CK13 and CK16, demonstrating a squamous transformation. The mesenchymal substance shows positive immunostaining for collagen IV, V, VI, and VII. Collagen II, aggrecan, and chondromodulin are present in chondroid-type areas.

Warthin tumor Cytologic preparations show lymphocytes, oncocytic cells, and a background of granular proteinaceous debris all present in variable proportions. The lymphocyte population usually is predominant and consists mainly of small cells mixed with a few larger lymphoid cells, plasma cells, mast cells, macrophages, and, sometimes, germinal center fragments. Oncocytic cells may be scant and usually form cohesive flat sheets, and in rare cases, they can be arranged in papillary or bilayered formations. The appearance of the oncocytic cytoplasm depends on the type of staining used: it appears granular, eosinophilic to gray–blue with Papanicolaou staining, whereas it appears dense, deep blue, and free of granules with May–Grünwald–Giemsa staining. Nuclei may be uniform, enlarged, round or oval, or eccentric or centrally placed, with distinct nucleoli. Squamous and/or mucinous metaplasia is frequently encountered.

The epithelial cells are immunoreactive for low-molecular-weight cytokeratins, EMA, and the secretory component. Some epithelial cells are positive for ribonuclease, lactoferrin, CEA, lysozyme, somatostatin, and MUC-2, whereas they are negative for S-100 protein, p63, calponin, actin, and GFAP. Lymphoid cells are positive for mature B-cell (CD20, CD79a, and PAX-5) and T-cell markers (CD2, CD3, CD4, CD5, CD7, and CD8). No light-chain restriction is present on B-lymphocytes.

Oncocytoma FNA smears show a discrete quantity of large polygonal cells with moderate to abundant, densely granular eosinophilic cytoplasm rich in mitochondria and small, round to oval, slightly eccentric or central nuclei with evident nucleoli. Oncocytes are arranged in flat sheets, cords, trabeculae, and papillary clusters. Moreover, some single cells can be seen. Immunocytochemistry shows positivity for CK7, CK8, CK18, CK19, and mitochondrial markers. Some cells can express CK14 and p63.

Basal cell adenoma Cytologic samples are cellular and show a variable amount of collagenous substance that appears basophilic metachromatic on May–Grünwald–Giemsa stain and brightly cyanophilic or eosinophilic on Papanicolaou stain. Numerous groups and branching cords composed of cohesive basaloid cells, sometimes with a peripheral palisading appearance, can be observed along with rare isolated cells and naked nuclei. The neoplastic cells are monomorphous with a small pale rim of cytoplasm and round to ovoid nuclei showing granular chromatin and occasionally distinct nucleoli. Immunocytochemical stains show positivity for CK7, CK8, CK18, CEA, and EMA. Some neoplastic cells are positive for CK5, CK14, S-100 protein, p63, CD10, calponin, and smooth muscle actin, demonstrating myoepithelial differentiation.

Canalicular adenoma This is a very rare, benign neoplasm, also known as ductal adenoma and typically located in the minor salivary glands, mainly in the lip. FNA specimens exhibit predominantly pseudopapillary clusters of bland-appearing columnar epithelial cells and small groups of round to oval or spindle-shaped basaloid cells with scant eosinophilic cytoplasm. The nuclei are round, and the chromatin is bland and finely granular with no evident nucleoli. Immunocytochemical stains show positivity for CK7, CK19, S-100 protein, and EMA. Some cells can express CD117, SOX-10, and GFAP, whereas myoepithelial markers are negative.

Sebaceous adenoma This rare benign neoplasm is composed of cohesive aggregates of epithelial cells showing sebaceous metaplastic changes with the characteristic finely vacuolated cytoplasm. Occasionally, the periphery of the epithelial clusters is surrounded by layers of basaloid cells. Foci of squamous metaplasia can be observed. The sebaceous cell differentiation is particularly evident in the air-dried cytologic preparation. In the presence of a large quantity of lymphoid cells, the correct diagnosis should be that of *sebaceous lymphadenoma*. The sebaceous cells express adipophilin, p63, EMA, D2-40, and XIIIa factor. The basaloid cells are positive for CK7 and occasionally for CD10.

Myoepithelioma The myoepithelial cells are identical to those of a pleomorphic adenoma, but the absence of mesenchymal substance and epithelial cells distinguishes it from a PA. Myoepithelial cells may exhibit spindle-shaped, plasmacytoid, epithelioid, and clear-cell features. These different cellular features can be seen in combination, but, often, one predominates, and then it can create a diagnostic challenge. Plasmacytoid myoepithelioma is the most frequent form and simulates a plasma cell lesion. A spindle cell myoepithelioma can be difficult to distinguish from tumors with a similar morphologic pattern, such as schwannoma or myofibroblastic tumor. The clear-cell variant can simulate other primitive neoplasms or metastatic deposits with clear-cell differentiation. Immunocytochemistry is helpful for identifying the myoepithelial cells, which are positive for CK7, CK14, p63, α-smooth muscle actin, and calponin. Immunoreactivity with S-100 protein, GFAP, and smooth muscle myosin heavy chain is variable.

Intraductal or ductal papilloma This is a rare lesion composed of cuboidal or columnar epithelial cells with abundant finely vacuolated cytoplasm and oval basally located nuclei, which are arranged in papillary structures with a fibrovascular core. The tumor cells are positive for CK7 and CK18 and are variably positive for CK19, vimentin, CEA, S-100 protein, and GCDFP-15.

4.3.4 Salivary Gland Carcinomas

Although malignant neoplasms of the salivary glands are less frequent than are benign lesions, when there is a clinical suspicion of malignancy, FNA is widely performed as part of the patient's preoperative management in view of the diagnostic utility. The parotid gland appears to be less commonly affected by malignant neoplasms than are the submandibular and minor salivary glands.

Mucoepidermoid carcinoma (MEC) Low-grade MEC is usually cystic and mucous-predominant (Fig. 4.45), whereas high-grade MEC is predominantly solid. FNA smears of low-grade MEC are often hypocellular and are characterized by a mixture of three epithelial cell types: squamous, intermediate epidermoid, and mucinous, all present in variable quantities in a background of mucoid material with cellular debris. Squamous cells are polygonal, with dense cyanophilic keratinized cytoplasm. The intermediate epidermoid cells form multilayered, tightly packed clusters, are smaller than squamous cells, and show a homogeneous, sharply outlined cytoplasm. The presence of cytoplasmic vacuoles may suggest a transition to mucus-secreting cells. Nuclei are small and round or oval, with a small nucleolus. Mucin-producing cells appear as columnar or signet-ring-like elements and show a large polyhedral vacuolated cytoplasm. Low-grade MEC has minimal nuclear atypia and may show glandular differentiation. Mucinous cells are positive for CK7, CK8 (Fig. 4.46), CK18, CK19, androgen receptors (Fig. 4.47), MUC-4, and MUC-5A. Squamous cells are immunostained with CK5, CK14, CK17, p63 (Fig. 4.48), and

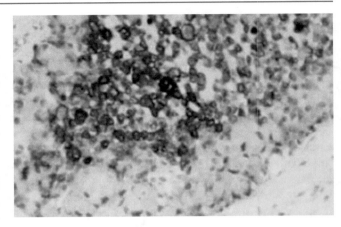

Fig. 4.46 Salivary gland mucoepidermoid carcinoma. CK8 immunostain (high magnification)

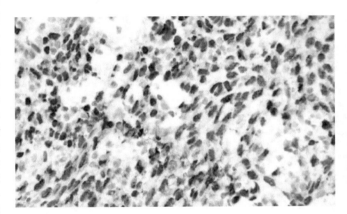

Fig. 4.47 Salivary gland mucoepidermoid carcinoma. Androgen receptor (AR) immunostain (high magnification)

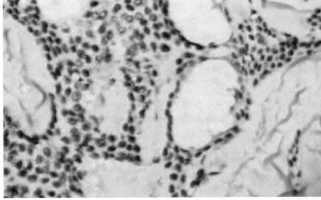

Fig. 4.48 Salivary gland mucoepidermoid carcinoma. p63 immunostain (high magnification)

EMA. In low-grade MEC, there is a translocation t(11;19)(q21;p13) involving the *MECT1* and *MAML2* genes. Nuclear immunostaining of the tumor with a specific antibody reveals the presence of MECT1–MAML2 fusion transcript.

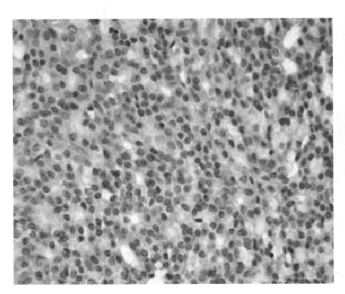

Fig. 4.45 Salivary gland mucoepidermoid carcinoma. Romanowsky stain (high magnification)

Acinic cell carcinoma FNA is usually cellular with single and haphazardly grouped cells, including the formation of acinar arrangements (Fig. 4.49) or even papillary fronds around a fibrovascular core. The cells are large and polygonal, with delicate, abundant, vacuolated, slightly basophilic to eosinophilic cytoplasm. Cytoplasmic vacuolization can be clearly observed on May–Grünwald–Giemsa stain, which also allows visualizing the presence of metachromatic zymogen granules. PAS-positive and diastase-resistant histochemical stain can be used for identifying the cytoplasmic zymogen granules. The nuclei are usually bland, round to oval, uniform, and eccentric, with small nucleoli commonly present. Nuclear pseudoinclusions can occasionally be seen. The presence of numerous naked nuclei and a granular background are the result of the fragility and friability of the cytoplasmic membrane. Most neoplastic cells express CK7, CK8, CK18, E-cadherin (Fig. 4.50), SOX-10 (Fig. 4.51), and DOG-1 (Fig. 4.52). Some tumor cells show positive immunocytochemical reactions for EMA, lactoferrin, α-1-antitrypsin, α-1-antichimotripsin, transferrin, CEA, Leu M1,

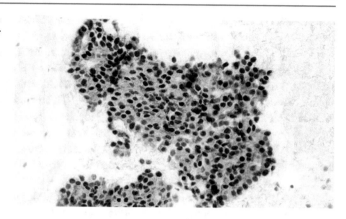

Fig. 4.51 Salivary gland acinic cell carcinoma. SOX-10 immunostain (high magnification)

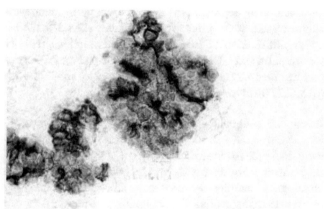

Fig. 4.52 Salivary gland acinic cell carcinoma. DOG-1 immunostain (high magnification)

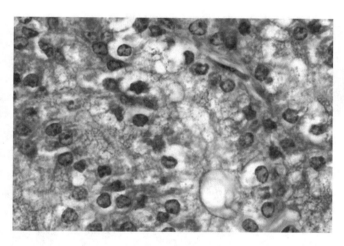

Fig. 4.49 Salivary gland acinic cell carcinoma. H&E stain (high magnification)

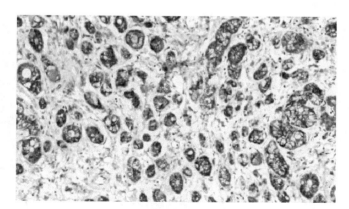

Fig. 4.50 Salivary gland acinic cell carcinoma. E-cadherin immunostain (high magnification)

COX2, p53, and bcl-2. Positivity for α-amylase and S-100 protein is not constant.

Adenoid cystic carcinoma Three different histologic variants (tubular, cribriform, and solid) have been described, although a mixed pattern is commonly seen cytologically. The tubular and cribriform variants are composed of small, oval basaloid cells, with scant and clear cytoplasm and hyperchromatic, often angulated nuclei with no evident nucleoli. In most samples, acellular matrix globules are visible as a metachromatic substance with May–Grünwald–Giemsa stain. FNA samples of the solid variant differ from the tubular and cribriform variants due to the predominance of basaloid cells and a lack of acellular matrix. Basaloid cells of the solid variant are usually arranged in three-dimensional clusters and show more cellular and nuclear pleomorphism than do the basaloid cells of the tubular and cribriform variants. Immunocytochemical reactions show the presence of two cell populations with distinct cellular immunophenotypes: epithelial and myoepithelial. Epithelial cells are positive for CK7, CK8, CK14, CK17, CK18, CK19, CEA, EMA, and CD117, whereas myoepithelial elements express CK5, CK14, CK17, CD43, vimentin, CD10, calponin, p63, actin, and S-100 protein. The t(6;9)(q22-23;p23-24) or the t(8;9) (q13;p22) translocation is detected in about 60% of adenoid cystic carcinomas, producing, respectively, MYB-NFIB and MYBL1-NFIB fusion transcripts. Immunocytochemistry for MYB overexpression is positive in almost all cases, even in the absence of a detectable translocation. Therefore, immunostaining for MYB can be used for diagnostic purposes.

Salivary gland clear-cell adenocarcinoma FNA cytology of this primary malignancy shows monotonous cells with moderate to abundant clear cytoplasm, well-defined cytoplasmic borders, and round and uniform nuclei with small nucleoli. The groups or sheets of neoplastic cells show ductal, but not myoepithelial, differentiation by immunocytochemistry and are positive for CK5, CK6, CK7, CK8, CK14, CK17, CK18, EMA, CEA, and p63. Occasionally, positivity for vimentin and GFAP is seen. The FISH test on FNA samples can be used for assessment of the translocation t(12;22) (q13;q12) involving the *EWSR1* and *ATF1* genes.

Basal cell adenocarcinoma This tumor is cytologically identical to basal cell adenoma; therefore, it is morphologically distinguishable from the latter, and the correct diagnosis is made only by certifying their infiltrative growth on histological samples. Furthermore, there are currently no markers that differentiate the benign form from its malignant counterpart.

Salivary duct adenocarcinoma FNA preparations show cell sheets and complex aggregates arranged in papillary, cribriform, and solid structures. Cells are polygonal with vacuolated or granular cytoplasm and hyperchromatic and pleomorphic nuclei with a prominent central nucleolus (Fig. 4.53). Background necrosis is usually present, and occasional psammoma bodies and squamous and/or oncocytic metaplasia may be seen. Characteristics of this tumor are the nuclear immunoreactivity for the androgen receptor (Fig. 4.54) and the membrane positivity for HER-2 (Fig. 4.55). Moreover, neoplastic cells show positivity for CK7 (Fig. 4.56), CK8, CK18, CK19, EMA CEA, LeuM1, p63 (Fig. 4.57), and gross cystic disease fluid protein-15 (GCDFP-15) (Fig. 4.58). Some cells also express CK5, CK14, and TAG B72.3.

Myoepithelial carcinoma The FNA cytology is similar to that of myoepithelioma. In fact, cases with a single cell type or with a mixture of plasmacytoid, spindle, epithelioid, stellate, and clear cells can be observed. Myoepithelial carcinoma may be distinguished from myoepithelioma by the presence of marked nuclear atypia, pleomorphism, coarse chromatin, and prominent nucleoli. A necrotic background

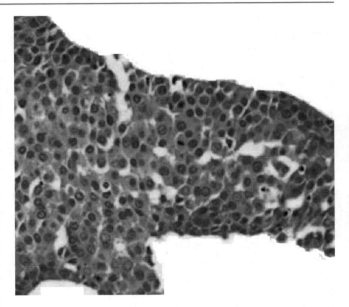

Fig. 4.53 Salivary gland duct cell carcinoma. H&E stain (high magnification)

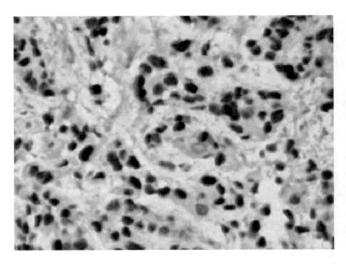

Fig. 4.54 Salivary gland duct cell carcinoma. Androgen receptor (AR) immunostain (high magnification)

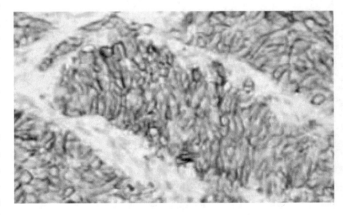

Fig. 4.55 Salivary gland duct cell carcinoma. HER-2 immunostain (high magnification)

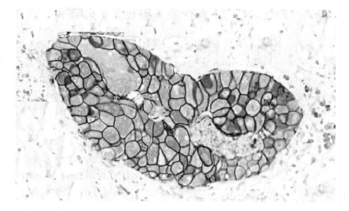

Fig. 4.56 Salivary gland duct cell carcinoma. CK7 immunostain (high magnification)

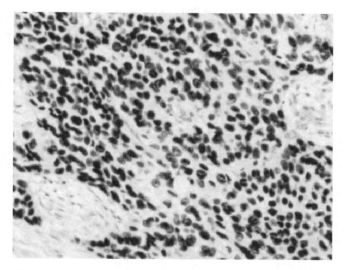

Fig. 4.57 Salivary gland duct cell carcinoma. p63 immunostain (high magnification)

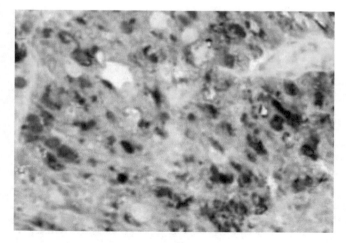

Fig. 4.58 Salivary gland duct cell carcinoma. GCDFP-15 immunostain (high magnification)

may be present. Neoplastic cells exhibit the myoepithelial immunophenotype and show reactivity for CK5, CK6, CK14, CK17, p63, α-SMA, calponin, smooth muscle myosin, S-100 protein, and CD10. In many cases, positivity for CK19 is also observed in some cells.

Epithelial–myoepithelial carcinoma Cytologic preparations usually show round groups or cellular aggregates of two different cell populations in a background that may contain abundant isolated clear cells and naked nuclei. One cell population consists of small, cuboidal duct-type epithelial cells with scant, dense, finely granular cytoplasm and large round to oval nuclei with a distinct nucleolus. The second cell population, which is often predominant, is composed of large polygonal myoepithelial cells that have an abundant glycogen-rich cytoplasm, enlarged oval or round vesicular nuclei with dispersed chromatin, and small distinct nucleoli. Epithelial cells express CK7, CK8, CK18, CK19, and EMA, whereas myoepithelial cells are positive for CD5, CK14, smooth muscular actin, p63, calponin, S-100 protein, and vimentin. Occasional CK17-immunopositive cells can be observed.

Carcinoma ex-pleomorphic adenoma The FNA cytologic diagnosis is often difficult because, usually, neoplastic cells are observed without the PA component; or only the elements of the benign lesion are present. The clinical history and a preexisting diagnosis of PA may suggest this diagnosis. Immunocytochemical stains can be extremely variable. An epithelial component is usually observed with positivity for CK7, CK8, CK18, and CK19 and myoepithelial cells expressing CK5, CK19, p63, vimentin, α-SMA, calponin, and S-100 protein.

Mammary analogue secretory carcinoma (MASC) FNA cytologic preparations show moderate to high cellularity, with dispersed or loosely cohesive cells arranged in sheets and clusters with a papillary, pseudopapillary, and/or an acinar-like configuration. Neoplastic cells have abundant vacuolated to granular eosinophilic cytoplasm, which is occasionally mucin-filled. Extracellular mucoid secretory material is present in the background. Cells show immunopositivity for CK7, CK8, CK18, CK19, EMA, vimentin, MUC1, MUC4, GATA3, STAT5a, GCDFP15, mammaglobin, and adipophilin. Moreover, FISH analysis shows translocation of the *ETV6* gene locus, forming ETV6-NTRK3 gene fusion.

Carcinosarcoma Cytologic preparations show pleomorphic duct epithelial carcinoma cells admixed with neoplastic mesenchymal cells. From the immunocytochemistry point of view, each component maintains its own immunophenotype as if it were present alone. Therefore, the carcinomatous portion expresses CK7, CK8, CK18, CK19, sometimes androgen receptors, and/or GCDFP-15, whereas the neoplastic mesenchymal component is immunoreactive for S-100 protein and collagen II or osteonectin, showing their chondrosarcoma or osteosarcoma nature.

Lymphoepithelial carcinoma FNA samples include a mixture of lymphoid cells, plasma cells, and neoplastic epithelial cells with pleomorphic, large or spindle cells, which are single or arranged in small sheets. Epithelial cells express CK5, CK8, CK13, CK19, p63, and p40, demonstrating their squamous differentiation. Lymphoid elements composed of B- and T-lymphocytes and lymphoplasmacytic and polyclonal plasma cells are numerous. The strong association with EBV is demonstrated by highlighting of the nuclear presence of viral nucleic acid by use of molecular in situ hybridization (EBER), whereas immunocytochemical positivity for LMP-1 is variable.

Squamous cell carcinoma FNA samples of this very rare primary neoplasm of the salivary glands show keratinizing or nonkeratinizing epithelial cells that are indistinguishable from those of metastatic squamous cell carcinoma or from atypical squamous metaplasia present in other salivary gland tumors. Currently, there are no immunocytochemical markers or biomolecular tests that are useful for differentiating primary from metastatic squamous carcinoma.

Oncocytic carcinoma This is another extremely rare carcinoma that causes pitfalls in FNA diagnosis, because it can easily be misinterpreted as oncocytoma or one of the other salivary gland lesions with oncocytic features. The presence of cells with abundant dense, granular cytoplasm, large nuclei with prominent nucleoli, marked cytologic atypia, mitotic activity, and necrosis in the clinical setting of rapid tumor growth, suspicious imaging studies, and facial nerve involvement must alert the physician to the possibility of an oncocytic carcinoma. Immunocytochemical positivity is the same as that for oncocytoma.

Poorly differentiated carcinoma The cytologic preparations can be similar to those of small-cell or large-cell carcinoma, usually with neuroendocrine features, and appears indistinguishable from the analogous carcinoma of the lung. FNA samples are hypercellular and are characterized by isolated and loosely cohesive clusters of cells with oval to round nuclei, dispersed granular chromatin, moderate pleomorphism, and indistinct or absent nucleoli. Focal nuclear molding is usually present. Neoplastic cells usually react with antibodies to neuroendocrine markers, such as CD56, NSE, synaptophysin, and chromogranin. Cytokeratin immunostaining shows the characteristic paranuclear dot-like pattern, and most primary small-cell carcinomas of the salivary gland (and Merkel cell carcinomas) show positivity for CK 20.

4.3.5 Primary Salivary Gland Lymphomas

Primary and secondary lymphomas can occur in the salivary glands, especially in the parotid gland. Most primary lymphomas are of the B-cell type, and the most common are MALT-type, follicular, and large B-cell lymphomas. Immunocytochemistry or flow cytometry is recommended for making a correct diagnosis.

MALT-type lymphoma FNA samples are composed of a mixed population of lymphoid cells, with an increased number of marginal-zone or monocytoid B cells, lymphoplasmacytes, plasmacytoid cells, scattered immunoblasts, and plasma cells (Figs. 4.59 and 4.60). In some cases, there is a predominance of plasmacytoid cells. Neoplastic cells are positive for CD19, CD20 (Fig. 4.61), CD45, PAX-5, and bcl-2, and they exhibit light-chain immunoglobulin monoclonality (Figs. 4.62 and 4.63).

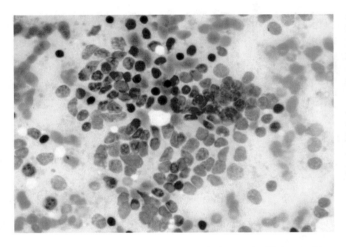

Fig. 4.59 Salivary gland MALToma. Papanicolaou stain (high magnification)

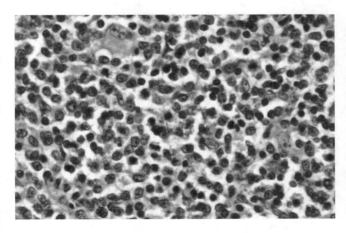

Fig. 4.60 Salivary gland MALToma. H&E stain (high magnification)

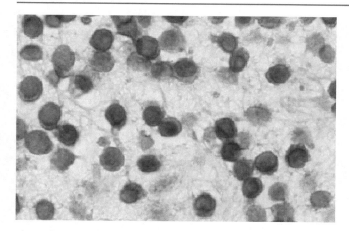

Fig. 4.61 Salivary gland MALToma. CD20 immunostain (high magnification)

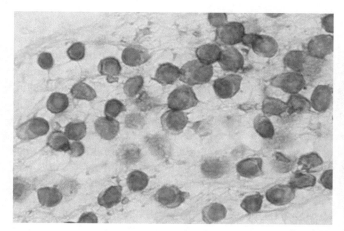

Fig. 4.62 Salivary gland MALToma. Lambda chain immunostain (high magnification)

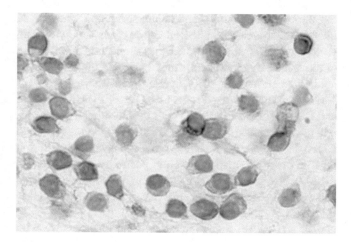

Fig. 4.63 Salivary gland MALToma. Kappa chain immunostain (high magnification)

Follicular cell lymphoma This mostly originates from peri-parotid lymph nodes rather than from the salivary glands. Variable amounts of centrocytes and centroblasts mixed with other lymphoid elements can be observed on FNA cytology preparations (Fig. 4.64). The neoplastic cells express CD10 (Fig. 4.65), CD19, CD20 (Fig. 4.66), CD79a, bcl-2, bcl-6, PAX-5, and monoclonal membrane light-chain immunoglobulin (Fig. 4.67).

Large-cell B-cell lymphoma FNA cytology smears are cellular and composed of centroblast-like cells and/or immunoblasts variably mixed with mature small lymphocytes, macrophages, and plasma cells. On flow cytometry methods or immunocytochemistry, the neoplastic cells show light-chain restriction and expression of surface CD20, CD79a, and PAX-5. Moreover, the GCB subtype is positive for CD10 and/or bcl-6 and/or bcl-2, whereas the ABC subtype expresses MUM-1.

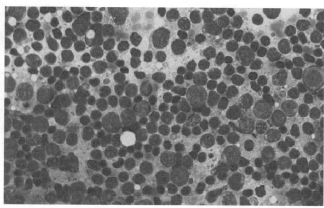

Fig. 4.64 Salivary gland follicular lymphoma. Romanowsky stain (high magnification)

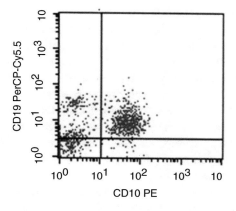

Fig. 4.65 Salivary gland follicular lymphoma. CD10/CD19 flow cytometry (high magnification)

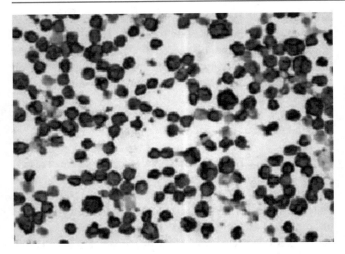

Fig. 4.66 Salivary gland follicular lymphoma. CD20 immunostain (high magnification)

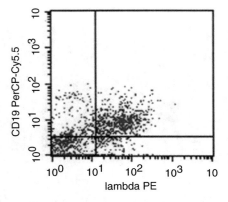

Fig. 4.67 Salivary gland follicular lymphoma. Lambda/CD19 flow cytometry (high magnification)

4.3.6 Metastases to the Salivary Glands

Secondary tumors of the salivary glands are not uncommon and mainly involve the parotid and major salivary glands. Sometimes the metastases affect the lymph nodes enclosed in the glandular parenchyma or lymph nodes adjacent to the gland instead of the glandular tissue. The origin of the primary site of the tumor is often in the head and neck and predominantly from skin squamous cell carcinoma or malignant melanoma and very rarely from sources such as nasopharyngeal or thyroid carcinoma. The clinical history of a synchronous or metachronous non-salivary-gland malignancy or a cytomorphology different from that of primary tumors of the salivary gland should lead one to consider the presence of a metastatic lesion. Metastases often retain many cytologic characteristics related to the primary tumor; and therefore, direct microscopic comparison with the cytologic features of the primary neoplasm is useful. It is also useful to perform immunocytochemical investigations according to the cyto-

morphologic features of the neoplastic lesion and the clinical history. Therefore, the immunostaining panels should include:

– TTF-1 and napsin-A for lung adenocarcinoma
– S-100 protein, HMB-45, and melan A/MART-1 for melanoma
– Thyroglobulin, TTF-1, and PAX-8 for thyroid carcinoma
– CK20 and CDX-2 for colorectal carcinoma
– GATA-3 and mammaglobin for breast cancer
– RCC and CD10 for renal cell carcinoma
– B- and T-lymphocytes markers for lymphomas.

4.4 Breast

4.4.1 Normal Breast

FNA samples of a non-lactating breast show fibroadipose stromal elements, some ductal cells, and rare or absent acinar cells. The ductal epithelial cells have a cuboidal to columnar shape, regular oval nuclei with evenly distributed chromatin, and inconspicuous or occasionally small, distinct, centrally placed nucleoli. The myoepithelial cells have a small, indistinct, and elongated cytoplasm and oval, dark nuclei. Acinar cells are rarely present in FNA smears of normal breast tissue. When present, these cells have cuboidal features and usually are arranged in small aggregates. Sometimes, small fragments of lobular units that are made up of acini incorporated in a bland stroma which also includes very small portions of terminal ducts can be observed in cytologic specimens. The luminal epithelial cells are cuboidal and/or cylindrical and are arranged in a single layer surrounded by myoepithelial elements. A basal lamina is present surrounding the terminal ductules and acinic structures. The size of the epithelial and myoepithelial cell nucleus and cytoplasm varies in relationship to the hormonal and functional phase of the mammary gland. In the luteal phase of the cycle, myoepithelial cells are enlarged, simulating histiocytes.

Acinar cells are usually positive for CK7, CK8, CK18, and CK19. The myoepithelial cells of interlobular and terminal ducts express CK5, CK14, CK17, p63, maspin, and CD10. The myoepithelial cells from the alveoli, in addition to the previous markers, show positivity for vimentin, α-SMA, heavy-chain immunoglobulin, smooth myosin, and calponin. The terminal duct cells have acinar and myoepithelial positivity that includes CK7, CK8, CK18, CK19, CK5, CK14, and CK17. Some ductal cells are also reactive with antibodies to maspin, CD10, and fatty acid synthase. The basal lamina can be highlighted by use of antibodies for vimentin, type IV collagen, and laminin. Furthermore, variable amounts of epithelial cells show positivity for estrogen and progesterone receptors (ER and PgR).

4.4.2 Benign Non-neoplastic Lesions

Most common breast benign non-neoplastic processes include cysts, fibrocystic change, mastitis, breast abscesses, fat necrosis, lactation changes, radiation change, fibroadenoma, and gynecomastia.

Simple mammary cysts FNA cytologic samples have poor cellularity, consisting mainly of foamy histiocytes; variable numbers of duct cells and apocrine cells, both single and gathered in small sheets; and debris in the background. Apocrine cells have abundant granular cytoplasm and round, centrally located nuclei with a prominent nucleolus. Marked enlargement of epithelial cells is observed in regenerative and reparative features. Immunohistochemical staining for CD68 can be used for demonstration of the histiocyte/macrophage nature of foam cells. Immunostaining for S-100 protein and CD1a is useful for distinguishing apocrine cells from a granular cell tumor (schwannoma) or Langerhans cell histiocytosis. Immunostaining for androgen receptors identifies apocrine cells.

Fibrocystic change This is a modification of breast tissue that includes dilation of the intralobular glands and connective tissue fibrosis, which may be associated with mild epithelial hyperplasia, apocrine metaplasia, and focal adenosis. FNA cytologic specimens are usually hypercellular and are composed of a mixture of various cell populations, including small fragments of adipose and connective tissue, sheets of ductal cells with honeycomb features, and interspersed myoepithelial cells, clusters and/or single apocrine cells, foamy macrophages, and cystic debris that is sometimes calcified. Immunocytochemistry can be used for identifying the different cell populations that show the immunopositivity of normal cells.

Mastitis FNA samples show different cell types, depending on the nature of the inflammation. Variable numbers of cohesive sheets of epithelial cells with well-maintained cell polarity and myoepithelial cells in the background are observed. Reactive and reparative cell changes, ranging from slight to intense, are present. A purulent smear pattern with abundant neutrophils, debris, histiocytes, and macrophages is usually present in *acute mastitis* (Fig. 4.68). Abundant amorphous and granular debris with lymphocytes, plasma cells, macrophages, and, sometimes, multinucleated giant histiocytes is observed in *chronic mastitis*. The cytologic samples of *granulomatous mastitis* are composed of granulomas of the foreign-body type, aggregates of epithelioid histiocytes, lymphocytes, plasma cells, and rare clusters of ductal cells. Histochemical or immunocytochemical stains and molecular biology tests must be performed for assessment of the presence of mycobacteria in tuberculosis-endemic areas when a

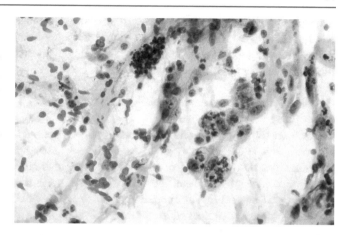

Fig. 4.68 Breast acute mastitis. Papanicolaou stain (high magnification)

necrotic caseous background and/or calcific deposits are present. *Idiopathic granulomatous mastitis* is a chronic inflammatory lesion of unknown etiology, which sometimes can simulate carcinoma both clinically and radiographically. Cytologic preparations show abundant cellularity composed of a mixture of chronic inflammatory cells with granulomatous tissue fragments including fibroblasts and epithelioid histiocytes that sometimes can mimic malignant ductal cells. Immunocytochemistry with CD68 and/or CD163 can be performed to confirm the histiocytic nature of the epithelioid cells.

Subareolar abscess This lesion, localized behind the nipple, is caused by inflammation due to squamous metaplasia of the lactiferous ducts, with consequent obstruction, dilatation, and rupture of the ducts. FNA cytology shows abundant cellularity consisting of acute and chronic inflammatory cells, some multinucleated giant cells of the foreign-body type, foamy histiocytes, nucleated and anucleated squamous cells, clusters of ductal cells, fragments of granulation tissue, and cholesterol crystals. Immunocytochemistry usually is not performed; however, in some cases proliferation markers can be used to exclude a neoplastic process.

Pregnancy and lactation Hormonal stimulation causes the lobular units of the terminal ducts to become hyperplastic and show cytoplasmic vacuolization in keeping with the secretory changes. Occasionally, the formation of a nodule, a *lactating adenoma*, can be observed. Cytologic preparations from FNA show high cellularity and numerous densely compressed acinar cell clusters with myoepithelial cells on the periphery. The immunocytochemical profile is similar to that of normal breast cells.

Fat necrosis This trauma-related inflammatory lesion is caused by necrosis of mammary or subcutaneous fatty tissue. FNA cytology usually shows scant epithelial cellularity, necrotic and degenerated adipocytes, foamy macrophages, and multinucleated foreign-body-type giant cells along with a few inflammatory cells (neutrophils, lymphocytes, and plasma cells). Immunocytochemical tests are usually of no value. Markers can occasionally be used for confirmation of the histiocytic/macrophage nature of epithelioid elements.

Gynecomastia This hormone (endogenous and exogenous)-related lesion is caused by a relative increment in estrogen activity, a decrease in androgen activity, or a combination of both, which causes hyperplasia and hypertrophy of connective mammary tissue and ductal epithelium in males. The FNA aspirate is sparsely cellular and is composed of monolayers of cohesive ductal epithelial cells, sometimes arranged in papillary-like fragments. Nucleolated cells with mild nuclear atypia as well as apocrine cells may occur. Epithelial cells show the same immunophenotype as do normal breast cells.

4.4.3 Benign Epithelial Proliferations

This section includes the different types of adenosis (sclerosing, apocrine, microglandular, radial scar/complex) and adenomas (tubular, lactating, apocrine, and ductal). A specific diagnosis of adenosis or adenoma cannot be made cytologically, and the FNA diagnosis of benign proliferative lesion should be made instead.

Adenosis FNA exhibits poor cellularity due to the significant stromal sclerosis that is present; smears show sheets of ductal epithelial cells, apocrine cells, numerous myoepithelial cell nuclei, macrophages, and stromal fragments. In adenosis, except in the microglandular type, the presence of myoepithelial cells may be highlighted with immunostain positivity for CK5, CK14, CK17, α-SMA, p63, and calponin. In microglandular adenosis, these markers are negative, whereas S-100 protein is positive.

Tubular adenoma Cytologic preparations are cellular, and cells are arranged in small, three-dimensional cohesive groups, tubules, and acini. No stromal fragments are observed, and naked nuclei are scarce. Single cells have a moderate amount of pale cytoplasm, regular nuclei, and inconspicuous nucleoli. Myoepithelial cells also appear in the epithelial cell groups. If present, the rare stromal cells are positive for CD34, bcl-2, and smooth muscle actin, demonstrating their myofibroblastic nature. Sometimes stromal cells can express PgR. Epithelial and myoepithelial cells show their typical immunophenotype. Epithelial cells are also positive for ER and PgR.

Lactating adenoma Cytologic samples show cohesive monolayers of enlarged monomorphic cells exhibiting round nuclei with prominent single nucleoli, abundant foamy cytoplasm, mild atypia, and a finely vacuolated/foamy background containing variable numbers of naked nuclei. The cytologic immunophenotype is comparable to that of normal breast cells.

Apocrine adenoma FNA cytology preparations may show two different types of apocrine cells. One type has eosinophilic granular cytoplasm and globoid nuclei with one or two prominent nucleoli. The other type has a foamy cytoplasm with small vacuoles containing lipofuscin pigment and central, round nuclei with one or two nucleoli. Apocrine cells are immunoreactive with CK8, CK18, EMA, GCDFP-15, apolipoprotein D, and α2-glycoprotein. They express androgen receptor, but no ER or PgR.

Ductal adenoma Cytologic samples show cohesive cell clusters consisting of luminal epithelial and myoepithelial cells, accompanied by occasional apocrine metaplastic cells. The immunocytochemistry is similar to that of normal mammary ducts. ER and PgR are expressed, but not HER-2.

4.4.4 Breast Carcinoma

Because cytomorphologic distinction between in situ and invasive carcinoma is not possible by FNA, the two forms of carcinoma are usually grouped together under the cytologic category of "breast carcinoma."

Ductal carcinoma FNA cytologic preparations are hypercellular and are composed of sheets and cords of crowded neoplastic cells with overlapping nuclei and irregular outlines (Figs. 4.69 and 4.70). Single tumor cells may show plasmacytoid features with hyperchromatic, minimally atyp-

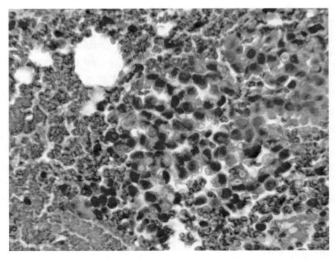

Fig. 4.69 Breast ductal cell carcinoma. H&E stain (high magnification)

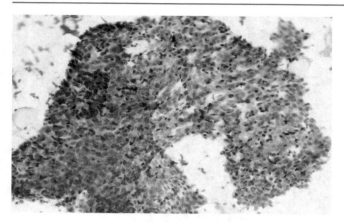

Fig. 4.70 Breast ductal cell carcinoma. Papanicolaou stain (high magnification)

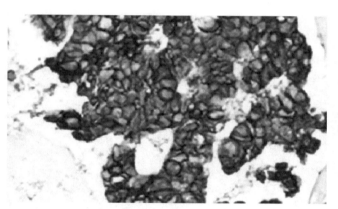

Fig. 4.71 Breast ductal cell carcinoma. CK7 immunostain (high magnification)

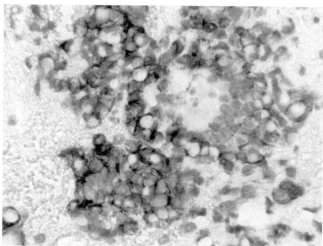

Fig. 4.72 Breast ductal cell carcinoma. E-cadherin immunostain (high magnification)

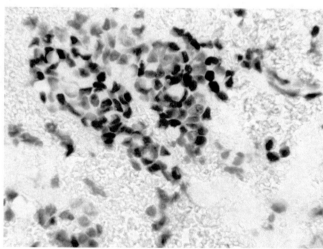

Fig. 4.73 Breast ductal cell carcinoma. ER immunostain (high magnification)

ical oval nuclei, including occasional prominent nucleoli in low-grade carcinoma. Single cells with pleomorphic, enlarged, and eccentric nuclei with marked contour irregularities and prominent nucleoli are present in high-grade carcinoma. Myoepithelial cells are absent. Most cases of ductal carcinoma exhibit the immunophenotypic pattern of "luminal"-type carcinomas, that is, expression of markers present in mammary duct cells: CK7 (Fig. 4.71), CK8, CK18, CK19, E-cadherin (Fig. 4.72), ER (Fig. 4.73), PgR (Fig. 4.74), and variable presence of HER-2 (Fig. 4.75).

Lobular neoplasia/carcinoma This term includes atypical lobular hyperplasia (ALH), lobular carcinoma in situ (LCIS), and invasive lobular carcinoma, because the cytomorphologic features usually overlap. FNA smears are usually hypocellular to moderately cellular and are composed of small, non-cohesive tumor cells with plasmacytoid features, round eccentric nuclei with fine chromatin, and inconspicuous nucleoli (Figs. 4.76 and 4.77). Some cells show intracytoplasmic vacuoles, each containing a mucinous globule. The pleomorphic variant of LCIS shows enlarged cells with

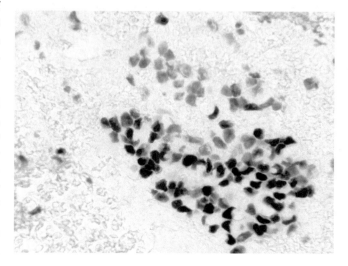

Fig. 4.74 Breast ductal cell carcinoma. PgR immunostain (high magnification)

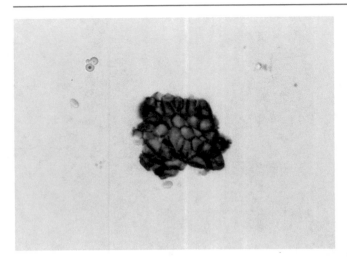

Fig. 4.75 Breast ductal cell carcinoma. HER-2 immunostain (high magnification)

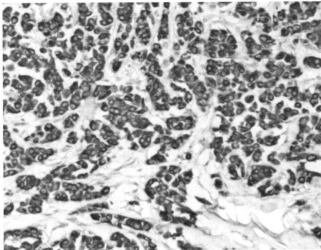

Fig. 4.78 Breast lobular carcinoma. CK7 immunostain (high magnification)

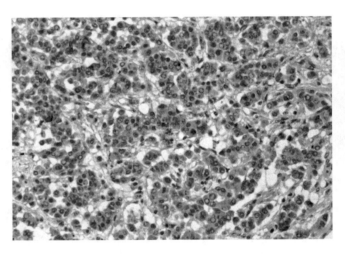

Fig. 4.76 Breast lobular carcinoma. H&E stain (high magnification)

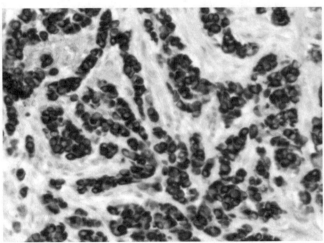

Fig. 4.79 Breast lobular carcinoma. CK19 immunostain (high magnification)

nuclear pleomorphism, prominent nucleoli, and abundant cytoplasm with apocrine features. Necrosis and mitosis can be observed. Neoplastic cells are positive for CK7 (Fig. 4.78), CK8, CK18, CK19 (Fig. 4.79), CK14, and/or CK17. E-cadherin is negative (Fig. 4.80), whereas cytoplasmic p120 protein is visible (Fig. 4.81). Lobular neoplasms of the breast have alterations in the *CDH1* gene, mapped to chromosome 16 (16p22.1), which encodes E-cadherin. The silencing of this gene results in the absence of E-cadherin production and therefore the negativity of the specific immunostaining. Instead, the gene mutations determine the production of abnormal E-cadherin, whose immunocytochemical finding is evidenced by atypical aspects of immunostaining:

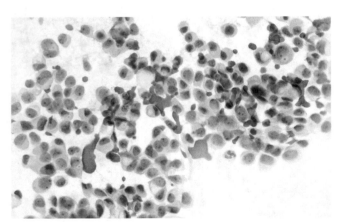

Fig. 4.77 Breast lobular carcinoma. Papanicolaou stain (high magnification)

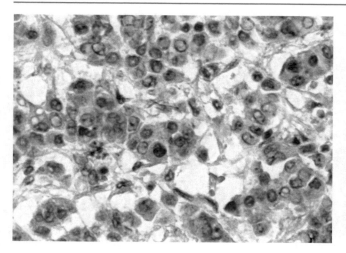

Fig. 4.80 Breast lobular carcinoma. E-cadherin CK7 immunostain (high magnification)

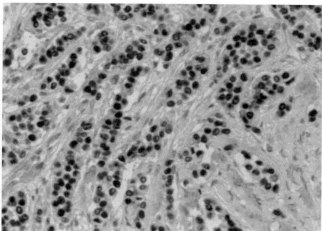

Fig. 4.82 Breast lobular carcinoma. ER immunostain (high magnification)

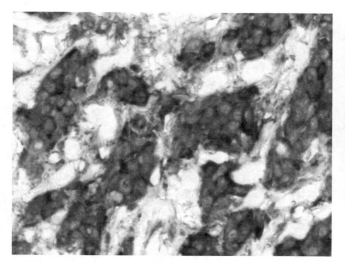

Fig. 4.81 Breast lobular carcinoma. p129 protein immunostain (high magnification)

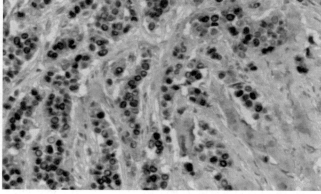

Fig. 4.83 Breast lobular carcinoma. PgR immunostain (high magnification)

the solubilization in the cytoplasm of the truncated protein results in cytoplasmic granulations, whereas the focal membrane or dot-like immunostaining is usually caused by protein synthesis abnormalities in its cytoplasmic portion. Most cases of lobular neoplasia are positive for ER (Fig. 4.82) and PgR (Fig. 4.83) and negative for HER-2. Pleomorphic LCIS usually is ER- and PgR-negative, whereas HER-2 is positive.

Tubular carcinoma Cytologic preparations show variable cellularity, with cohesive, uniform small cells arranged in sheets, small aggregates, and long tubules. Myoepithelial cells, stromal fragments, and naked nuclei are rare or absent. Neoplastic cells are positive for CK7, CK8, CK18, CK19,

and E-cadherin, whereas ER and PgR are almost always positive. Negative immunostainings are observed with HER-2, EGF-R, CK5/6, and CK14.

Mucinous carcinoma FNA cytology shows variable cellularity, with cohesive groups of monomorphic tumor cells having low-grade nuclear atypia often arranged in ball-like three-dimensional clusters surrounded by mucinous material. *Mucocele-like lesion*, a rare breast lesion that occurs in young patients, needs to be distinguished from mucinous carcinoma. This is done most reliably on resected specimens. Mucinous carcinoma shows low-molecular-weight cytokeratins and strong immunoreactivity for MUC-2, ER, and PgR. HER-2 is always negative, whereas variable numbers of neoplastic cells can express WT-1 and neuroendocrine markers.

Medullary carcinoma This diagnosis should not be formulated on cytologic preparations, but should only be hypothesized in the presence of high-grade cellular atypia, numerous lymphocytes, and plasma cells. FNA samples are usually hypercellular, consisting of syncytially arranged sheets of poorly differentiated large epithelial cells with enlarged nuclei and multiple irregular macronucleoli. Single neoplastic cells with high-grade atypia, naked large nuclei, lymphocytes, plasma cells, and occasional necrosis may be seen in the background. The immunophenotype of neoplastic epithelial cells is characterized by positivity for CK5, CK8, CK14, CK18, caveolin 1, β-catenin, and E- and P-cadherin. These tumors are often "triple negative" (absence of ER, PR, and HER2). Most cases express EGF-R and mutated *TP53*.

Apocrine carcinoma FNA cytology shows large single polygonal neoplastic cells, combined with loose groups or syncytial arrangements, showing an abundant granular eosinophilic cytoplasm, large hyperchromatic nuclei, and prominent nucleoli. The neoplastic cells express CK8, CK18, CD24, androgen receptors, GCDFP-15 (gross cystic disease fluid protein 15), TAG B72.3, 15-PDGH (prostaglandin dehydrogenase), ACMS1 (acyl-CoA synthase medium-chain family member 1), and GGT-1 (gamma-glutamyl transferase 1). ER and PgR are almost always negative, whereas about half of the cases have HER-2 and EGF-R overexpression.

Metaplastic breast carcinoma A group of neoplasias that includes adenosquamous carcinoma, carcinosarcoma (homologous or heterologous), and spindle cell carcinoma is comprised under this term. The cytologic features depend on the specific subtype of carcinoma and may be monomorphic or polymorphic that reflects the tumor composition: adenocarcinoma cells and neoplastic squamous epithelium, neoplastic spindle cells with an admixture of multinucleated giant cells, and/or heterologous neoplastic elements. Inflammatory cells, necrosis, and debris may be observed in the background. Immunocytochemistry reveals the nature of neoplastic cells: in *adenosquamous carcinoma*, the neoplastic cells express CK5, CK14, CK17, and p63 and in some cells CK7. In *carcinosarcoma*, the epithelial component shows positivity for EMA, vimentin, and CK7 and CK5 in occasional cells. The sarcomatous elements may express smooth muscle actin, myogenin, collagen II, S-100 protein, or osteonectin, depending on their smooth muscle, striated-muscle, chondroid, or osteochondroid origin. Immunocytochemistry in *spindle cell carcinoma* usually shows positivity for vimentin, CK7, CK14, and p63. All subtypes of metaplastic carcinoma show a triple-negative molecular profile, and most of them express EGF-R.

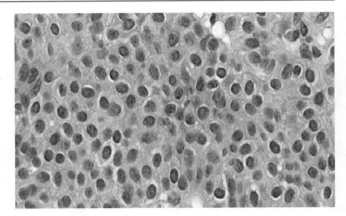

Fig. 4.84 Breast neuroendocrine tumor. H&E stain (high magnification)

Neuroendocrine tumor/carcinoma Three different entities are considered in this group: well-differentiated neuroendocrine tumor (carcinoid-like), poorly differentiated/small-cell neuroendocrine carcinoma, and invasive carcinoma with neuroendocrine differentiation. *Well-differentiated neuroendocrine tumors* are composed of single and crowded plasmacytoid cells with eccentric nuclei and a moderate amount of eosinophilic granular cytoplasm (Fig. 4.84). *Small-cell neuroendocrine carcinoma* shows cytologic features similar to those of other anatomic sites. Neuroendocrine differentiation has been demonstrated in up to 30% of invasive ductal carcinomas and is most frequently found in mucinous carcinomas, particularly the hypercellular variant, and in solid papillary carcinomas. The neoplastic cells demonstrate strong expression of CK8, CK18, CK19, chromogranin A (Fig. 4.85), synaptophysin (Fig. 4.86), CD56, and NSE. Most well-differentiated and poorly differentiated neuroendocrine tumors have a luminal A molecular profile, such as ER (Fig. 4.87) and PgR (Fig. 4.88)-positive and HER-2-negative.

Secretory carcinoma The cytologic preparations are cellular and show grape-like clusters of neoplastic cells, loosely cohesive clustered neoplastic cells, and single large cells with foamy, granular, or vacuolated cytoplasm, uniform round nuclei, slight nuclear pleomorphism, prominent nucleoli, and a mucinous background. Neoplastic cells show immunopositivity for CK5/6, CK8, CK14, CK18, S-100 protein, lactalbumin, and EGF-R, whereas CK7 is negative. The tumor is also negative for ER, PgR, and HER-2. There is a chromosomal translocation t(12;15)(q13;q25) that can be identified by FISH analysis done in FNA material. The fusion gene produces a chimeric protein that can be highlighted with ETV-6 antibody.

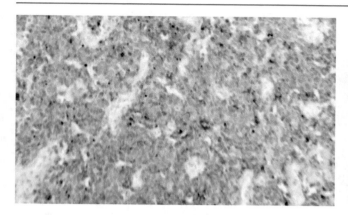

Fig. 4.85 Breast neuroendocrine tumor. Chromogranin A immunostain (medium magnification)

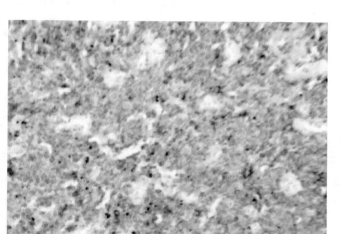

Fig. 4.86 Breast neuroendocrine tumor. Synaptophysin immunostain (medium magnification)

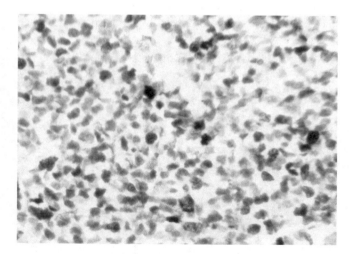

Fig. 4.87 Breast neuroendocrine tumor. ER immunostain (medium magnification)

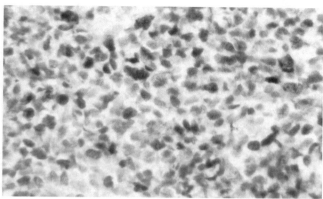

Fig. 4.88 Breast neuroendocrine tumor. PgR immunostain (medium magnification)

4.4.5 Epithelial/Myoepithelial Tumors

Biphasic epithelial and myoepithelial proliferations, such as pleomorphic adenoma and adenomyoepithelioma, are included in this group.

Pleomorphic adenoma The FNA cytology pattern is similar to that of the analogous tumor of the salivary glands: cohesive aggregates of epithelial cells admixed with fascicles of spindle stromal mesenchymal tissue and myoepithelial cells present in a myxoid matrix. Immunocytochemical staining displays the epithelial cells as positive for CK 7, whereas the myoepithelial cells are positive for CK5, CK6, CK14, CK17, p63, α-SMA, calponin, and S-100 protein. Antibodies to collagen IV stain the mesenchymal matrix and those for collagen II highlight the presence of chondroid-like areas.

Adenomyoepithelioma FNA smears are variably cellular, usually moderate to marked. Fragments of cohesive epithelial cells mixed with myoepithelial cells can be observed in varying proportions, even if the cellular distinction is rarely appreciated within the same fragment. The background shows cells with clear vacuolated cytoplasm and naked bipolar nuclei. Epithelial cells express low-weight cytokeratin, whereas myoepithelial markers such as CK5, CK6, CK14, CK17, p63, α-SMA, calponin, CD10, maspin, and S-100 protein are positive in myoepithelial cells.

Adenoid cystic carcinoma FNA cytology samples are characterized by the presence of crowded groups and spheres composed of a population of basaloid cells surrounding a globular matrix material. Immunocytochemistry highlights the basal/myoepithelial cells by their positivity to p63, calponin, smooth muscle actin, CK 5/CK6, and CK14. Epithelial cells express CK7, CK8, CK18, and CD117. Neoplastic cells are usually ER-, PgR- and HER2-negative, whereas EGFR overexpression is present in most cases.

4.4.6 Papillary Lesions

Papillary lesions of the breast include intraductal papilloma/papillomatosis, intracystic papillary carcinoma, solid papillary carcinoma, and micropapillary carcinoma.

Solitary (central) papilloma and papillomatosis *Papilloma* originates from the large ducts and usually develops in the areolar area, whereas *papillomatosis* (multiple or peripheral papillomas) develops from the terminal duct lobular units. They all share the same cytomorphologic aspects. FNA cytologic preparations are composed of three-dimensional and flat cell clusters and papillary and pseudopapillary fragments of epithelial and myoepithelial cells, with or without fibrovascular cores. Stripped nuclei, histiocytes, macrophages, atypical ductal epithelial cells, and apocrine cells may be seen. Immunostains reveal positivity for myoepithelial cells (smooth muscle myosin, calponin, maspin, p63, CK5/6, and CK14) and for epithelial cells (CK7, CK8, CK18, and CK19). Patchy positivity for ER and PgR is also present.

Intracystic (encapsulated) papillary carcinoma and intraductal papillary carcinoma The two show an identical cytomorphology; therefore, their distinction is not possible by FNA. Furthermore, FNA cytology cannot distinguish with certainty between papilloma and intracystic papillary carcinoma, particularly when there is mild to moderate cellular atypia. Cytologic samples are hypercellular and consist of crowded aggregates of tumor cells, some cellular fragments with papillary cores of stromal tissue, as well as pseudopapillary fronds. Low- to high-grade atypia is observed. Foamy histiocytes and macrophages are often present, whereas myoepithelial cells are absent. Immunoreactions with myoepithelial markers are negative. Strong positive immunostaining for ER is observed.

Solid papillary carcinoma FNA preparations are usually hypercellular and show fragments of small- to large-sized cells with a plasmacytoid-like or neuroendocrine appearance. The neoplastic cells have a granular eosinophilic cytoplasm, monotonous eccentric nuclei with bland fine chromatin, and inconspicuous nucleoli. The tumor cells are positive for low-molecular-weight cytokeratins, ER, and PgR. Some cells are positive for neuroendocrine markers and/or mucinous proteins.

Micropapillary carcinoma Cytologic samples are variably cellular and show neoplastic cells arranged in small and cohesive oval/round/angulated papillary structures, with or without a central fibrovascular core. Multinucleated and apocrine cells may be seen. Cell block sections may show epithelial cells surrounded by clear spaces and thin fibrous septa. Immunocytochemistry is analogous to that of solid papillary carcinoma. EMA immunostaining appears restricted to the basal portion of the neoplastic cells.

4.4.7 Mesenchymal Tumors

Potentially, every type of benign and malignant mesenchymal tumor can occur in the breast. The most frequent mesenchymal neoplasms are granular cell tumor, schwannoma, lipoma, myofibroblastoma, angiosarcoma, and liposarcoma.

Granular cell tumor FNA usually yields a sample with variable cellularity, composed of single or grouped large polygonal cells with granular cytoplasm and slight pleomorphic nuclei, often with prominent nucleoli. Cells show positive staining with S-100 protein and variable expression of CD68.

Schwannoma Cytologic specimens obtained by FNA may be paucicellular and show palisaded spindle cells that have the typical spindly or oval pleomorphic nuclei with homogeneous fine chromatin (Fig. 4.89). The neoplastic cells are immunoreactive with vimentin, S-100 protein (Fig. 4.90), calcineurin, CD56, CD57, and bcl-2. Calretinin, basic myelin protein, NGF-R, and CD99 show variable positivity.

Lipoma FNA cytology almost exclusively shows groups of uniform ballooned adipocytes and fragments of normal adipose tissue. Rare epithelial ductal cells, myoepithelial cells, and naked nuclei may be present. Normal adipocytes have

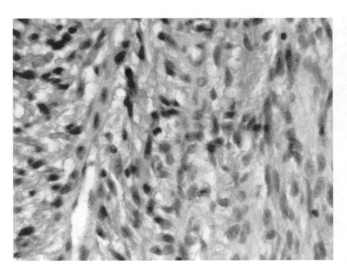

Fig. 4.89 Breast schwannoma. H&E stain (high magnification)

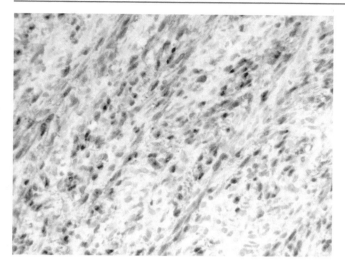

Fig. 4.90 Breast schwannoma. S-100 protein immunostain (high magnification)

positivity for vimentin, S-100 protein, and leptin; however, immunocytochemistry is not necessary for a diagnosis.

Myofibroblastoma This is subdivided into different subtypes. Predominant monomorphic spindle-shaped cells with oval or spindle nuclei with finely granular chromatin and absence of nucleoli characterize the *fibrous variant*. A variable amount of hyalinized collagen, often with a thread-like appearance, separates intersecting bundles of thin, bipolar, and uniform tumor cells. An occasional epithelioid cell population may be present focally. The *epithelioid subtype* exhibits single, loosely cohesive, and clustered oval tumor cells with granular cytoplasm and oval, bland nuclei; these cells are sometimes pleomorphic and binucleated, with grooves and intranuclear pseudoinclusions. Myofibroblastomas usually are diffusely immunoreactive for vimentin and have variable reactivity for desmin, calponin, smooth muscle actin, CD10, CD34, bcl-2, H-caldesmon, and CD99. Usually, ER, PgR, and androgen receptor positivity are detected.

Angiosarcoma The cytomorphologic aspects depend on the tumor grading. In FNA, *high-grade mammary angiosarcoma* shows single and loosely cohesive clusters of pleomorphic malignant round, oval, or spindle cells, in a focal ill-defined acinar or trabecular arrangement, in a bloody background that may also contain inflammatory cells, macrophages, and adipocytes. In *low-grade angiosarcoma*, monotonous slightly atypical single cells, thick three-dimensional branching aggregates, and papillary tufts may be observed. Sometimes, the cell aggregates reveal small arborizing thin-walled blood vessels. The neoplastic cells express CD31, CD34, Fli-1, ERG, HIF-1a, vascular endothelial growth factor (VEGF), and its receptor (VEGF-R) on immunostaining. Focal positivity for Factor VIII-related antigen is usually present, whereas ER and PgR are absent. *Epithelioid angiosarcoma* cells frequently express EMA and low-molecular-weight cytokeratins.

Liposarcoma Cytologic specimens obtained by FNA demonstrate variable cellularity of atypical cells that occur singly and in small groups. The cell morphology varies from spindly to round or polygonal, with hyperchromatic nuclei containing coarse chromatin and occasional nucleoli. Immunocytochemical staining is usually positive for MDM-2 and CDK4 in the various subtypes of liposarcoma. Atypical adipose tissue tumors express S-100 protein, whereas desmin and myogenin are usually present in dedifferentiated liposarcoma, and CD34 is found in the myxoid subtype.

4.4.8 Fibroepithelial Tumors

Belonging in this group, the WHO considers fibroadenoma, benign and malignant phyllodes tumor, and hamartoma.

Fibroadenoma The cytologic preparations are usually hypercellular and often show folded sheets of cohesive ductal epithelial cells, branches with a "papillary," finger-like branching, staghorn-like structures, or even tubule formations. Sometimes clusters of ductal cells with a "honeycomb" appearance are present. Cells or nuclei of myoepithelial elements are observed within and at the periphery of epithelial cell groups. Fragments of stromal tissues, apocrine cells, and foamy and giant histiocytes may be present. Epithelial cells are positive for CK7, CK8, CK18, and CK19, whereas myoepithelial cells express p63. Variable amounts of epithelial cells show positivity for ER and PgR. A positive androgen receptor stain identifies apocrine cells. Stromal elements can be stained with CD34 and/or α-SMA.

Phyllodes tumors These are also biphasic tumors, showing epithelial and stromal proliferation, but with a more pronounced stromal cellularity than that found in fibroadenomas. Histologically, phyllodes tumors are classified as benign, borderline, or malignant. This distinction can only be suspected, but cannot be diagnosed by cytology. FNA is usually hypercellular and shows mildly cohesive epithelial cells arranged in large, sometimes folded fragments admixed with abundant large, sometimes atypical, cohesive, and dispersed spindle cells. In *malignant phyllodes tumors,* there is greater cellularity, and the stromal elements acquire a sarcomatoid appearance. Immunocytochemistry shows the typical epithelial and myoepithelial markers, including hormone receptors like those seen in ductal cells. Neoplastic stromal cells are usually labeled with antibodies for vimentin, CD34, and collagen types I and III, and they have positive foci for endothelin (TE-1), bcl-2, CD117, EGFR, and the beta fraction of ER. No significant differences are observed between the benign and the malignant lesions, except that the latter show a greater percentage of MIB-1-positive cells.

Hamartoma Cytologic samples usually show moderate cellularity and are composed of two cellular components: epithelial and mesenchymal. There are acinar cells, ductal cells, and occasional apocrine, myoepithelial, and foam cells. Adipose tissue and isolated naked nuclei are present in variable amounts. Cytologic atypia is absent. The immunocytochemistry is comparable to that of the normal breast.

4.4.9 Lymphoma of the Breast

Any type of primary or secondary lymphoma may occur in the breast, and the cytologic findings are similar to those of lymphomas in other anatomic sites. Most primary lymphomas are of the B-cell type; the most common are small B-lymphocytic lymphoma, extranodal marginal-zone lymphoma (MALT-type), follicular lymphoma, and large B-cell lymphoma. A characteristic feature is the anaplastic large-cell lymphoma that is associated with breast prosthesis. Hodgkin lymphoma may also involve the breast tissue and usually is secondary. Flow cytometry and immunocytochemistry are necessary for demonstration of monoclonality and for providing the lymphoma subtype when lymphoma is suspected based on clinical findings and cytomorphology. Moreover, tissue biopsy is usually required for confirmation of the diagnosis.

Small B-lymphocytic lymphoma FNA samples are composed of numerous monotonous small lymphocytes with scant cytoplasm and round, uniform nuclei. Neoplastic cells are positive for CD5, CD19, CD20, CD45, PAX-5, and bcl-2 and show cytoplasmic membrane light-chain immunoglobulin monoclonality.

Extranodal marginal cell lymphoma Cytologic samples show a mixed lymphoid cell population composed of marginal-zone or monocytoid B cells, lymphoplasmacytes, plasmacytoid cells, scattered immunoblasts, and plasma cells (Fig. 4.91). The neoplastic cells are positive for CD19, CD20 (Fig. 4.92), CD45, PAX-5, and bcl-2 and have light-chain immunoglobulin monoclonality.

Follicular center cell lymphoma A mixed cell population of small, usually indented, lymphocytes and large lymphoid cell of the follicle center cell type characterizes this lymphoma. Distinction between follicular and diffuse growth patterns cannot be assessed on FNA cytology. The neoplastic cells express CD10, CD19, CD20, CD79a, bcl-2, bcl-6, PAX-5, and monoclonal membrane light-chain immunoglobulin.

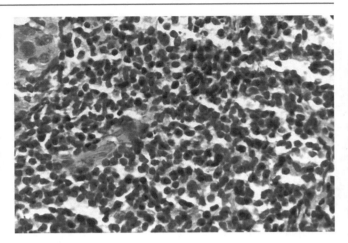

Fig. 4.91 Breast MALToma. H&E stain (high magnification)

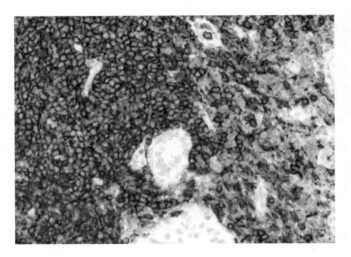

Fig. 4.92 Breast MALToma. CD20 immunostain (high magnification)

Large-cell B-cell lymphoma On cytologic preparations, centroblast-like cells and/or immunoblasts variously admixed with mature small lymphocytes, macrophages, and plasma cells may be observed. With use of flow cytometry methods or immunocytochemistry, the neoplastic cells show immunoglobulin light-chain restriction and expression of surface CD20, CD79a, and PAX-5. The GCB subtype is positive for CD10 and/or bcl-6 and/or bcl-2, whereas the ABC subtype expresses MUM-1.

Hodgkin lymphoma FNA cytology shows large cells with pale cytoplasm; two or more eccentrically placed large, complex, or lobulated nuclei exhibiting irregular borders; and eosinophilic macronucleoli (Reed–Sternberg cells) in a background of reactive mature small lymphocytes, plasma cells, immunoblasts, and variable numbers of eosinophils. These neoplastic cells express CD15, CD30, PAX-5, and occasionally bcl-6 and MUM-1.

Primary anaplastic (T-cell) lymphoma This usually arises as a mass around breast prosthesis. FNA cytology shows large cells with abundant dense cytoplasm and irregular, often polylobated and sometimes horseshoe-shaped nuclei containing prominent nucleoli (Fig. 4.93). Neoplastic cells are positive for CD2 (Fig. 4.94), CD4, CD30 (Fig. 4.95), and EMA, whereas ALK-1 is typically negative.

4.4.10 Metastases to the Breast

Metastases to the breast are rare. The most common primary sites include melanoma, lymphoma, and carcinoma of the lung, kidney, urogenital and gynecologic tract, and sarcomas.

The cytomorphology and immunocytochemistry usually agree with those of the primary tumor.

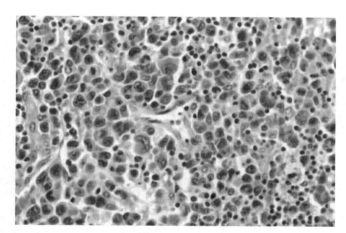

Fig. 4.93 Breast anaplastic lymphoma. H&E stain (high magnification)

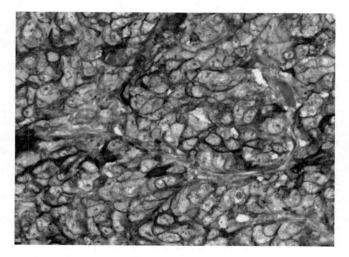

Fig. 4.94 Breast anaplastic lymphoma. CD2 immunostain (high magnification)

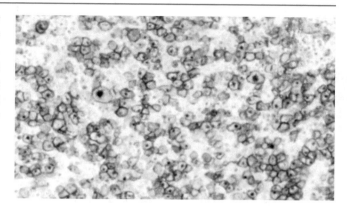

Fig. 4.95 Breast anaplastic lymphoma. CD30 immunostain (high magnification)

4.5 Lymph Node

FNA cytology of a lymph node has high cytomorphologic sensitivity and specificity for distinguishing between a benign lesion and a metastatic neoplasia. Regarding the diagnosis of lymphomatous lesions, the use of flow cytometry (preferred) or immunocytochemistry plays a fundamental role in the diagnosis and classification. We must emphasize that these ancillary tests complement and support the cytologic diagnosis of lymphoma.

4.5.1 Normal Lymph Node

The cytologic FNA preparations of the normal lymph node consist of a heterogeneous population of lymphoid elements: (1) small lymphocytes with scant cytoplasm and a round nucleus with coarsely textured chromatin; (2) follicular center cells of medium size with scant cytoplasm and irregular or cleaved nuclei with inconspicuous nucleoli (centrocytes); (3) follicular center large cells with scant basophilic cytoplasm and round, vesicular nuclei with one to three peripheral nucleoli placed close to the nuclear membrane (centroblasts); (4) large cells with moderate to abundant, clear or basophilic cytoplasm, round nuclei with fine, open chromatin, and one centrally located prominent nucleolus (immunoblasts); (5) macrophages with tingible bodies, voluminous cytoplasm filled with debris, a round or ovoid nucleus with finely granular chromatin, and a small or inconspicuous nucleolus; (6) interdigitating dendritic cells which are spindle-shaped, usually with abundant weakly eosinophilic cytoplasm and a spindle or ovoid nucleus, sometimes indented or double; (7) dendritic follicular cells which are ovoid or spindle-shaped and tend to aggregate, forming bundle, spiral, or storiform structures.

The small lymphocytes are partly B cells expressing CD19, CD20, and PAX-5 and partly T-lymphocytes, which are positive for CD2, CD3, CD4 or CD8, CD5, and CD7. Follicular center cells show positivity for CD10, CD19, CD20, PAX-5, and bcl-6. Macrophages may be identified by use of CD68. Interdigitating dendritic cells express vimentin, S-100 protein, fascin, and sometimes CD68 and lysozyme, whereas dendritic follicular cells are positive for vimentin, clusterin, desmoplakin, fascin, EGF-R, and HLA-DR; occasionally they express CD21, CD23, CD35, CNA.42, and KiM4p.

4.5.2   Reactive Follicular and Paracortical Hyperplasia

This is the response of the lymph node to an antigenic stimulus that results in the proliferation of certain areas of lymphoreticular tissue.

The cytologic pattern of follicular hyperplasia is related to the B-cell immune response and consists of variable amounts of small B-lymphocytes, T cells, centroblasts, centrocytes, immunoblasts, plasmacytic lymphocytes, plasma cells, histiocytes, and tingible-body macrophages.

On the other hand, paracortical hyperplasia is related to a T-cell response. Usually, predominant B-immunoblasts are admixed with a heterogeneous population of lymphoid cells, fragments of germinal centers containing centrocytes, centroblasts, dendritic cells, small lymphocytes, and tingible-body macrophages.

In reactive hyperplasia, B- and T-lymphocytes express normal markers, without immunoglobulin light-chain restriction or T-cell receptor rearrangement.

4.5.3   Benign Lymphadenopathies

These represent an increment in the volume of the lymph node, with persistence of normal architecture, caused by the proliferation of one or more populations of lymphoreticular tissue following an inflammatory/infectious process.

Acute bacterial lymphadenopathy FNA smears are very cellular and exhibit a purulent material that is composed almost exclusively of a population of variably degenerated neutrophils mixed with rare lymphocytes, plasma cells, and histiocytes. A portion of the purulent material should be submitted for culture studies. Immunocytochemistry studies usually are not helpful.

Cat scratch disease This infection is caused by a proteobacterium (*Bartonella henselae*). Cytologic preparations usually show clusters of epithelioid histiocytes enclosed by numerous neutrophils. Sometimes, the presence of numerous granulocytes may mask the presence of small granulomas. In many cases, microbiologic and/or serologic tests are required for formulation of the correct diagnosis, because other microorganisms, such as *Francisella tularensis* (which causes tularemia), *Chlamydia trachomatis* (which causes lymphogranuloma venereum), *Yersinia enterocolitica*, or *Y. pseudotuberculosis*, certain fungi, and, less commonly, *Mycobacterium tuberculosis* can also yield similar cytomorphologic features.

Mycobacterial infection FNA cytology usually shows granulomas with necrosis, sometimes necrosis only, or, less commonly, granulomas without necrosis. Only loose aggregates of histiocytes rather than true granulomas may be observed in immunocompromised patients. Special histochemical stains (alcohol-acid-fast stain) and immunocytochemistry for mycobacteria have low sensitivity; therefore, molecular techniques must be used for detecting mycobacterial infections.

Fungal lymphadenopathy FNA shows variable cellularity and various cellular compositions. In some cases, one can observe only a pure neutrophilic infiltrate; in other cases, only granulomas are present or a mixture of the two. Sometimes, only the fungal organisms are present, with few inflammatory cells. Culture tests and histochemical staining with periodic acid-Schiff (PAS), Grocott, and mucicarmine often allow the identification of the pathologic organism. Immunostaining with specific antibodies can also be used for identifying the fungal organism.

Infectious mononucleosis Cytologic samples contain numerous small lymphocytes mixed with variable numbers of immunoblasts, lymphoplasmacytes, some centroblasts, and a few plasma cells. Sometimes, large Reed–Sternberg-like cells or Hodgkin-like cells may be observed. Immunocytochemistry shows B-cell immunostaining positivity, an altered CD4/CD8 ratio, EBV antigens, and EBER positivity. Flow cytometry shows polyclonality.

Human immunodeficiency virus (HIV)-associated lymphadenopathy FNA alone does not yield an etiologic diagnosis of this process. The cytologic diagnosis of HIV-associated lymphadenopathy may be suspected only on the basis of clinical and serologic findings, because the follicular hyperplasia pattern present in the early stage of the disease is not specific. Likewise, the cytologic preparations are not useful for identifying Castleman-like features, lymphocyte depletion, follicular involution, or paracortical vascular hyperplasia present in the various phases of the disease. Immunocytochemistry only may be helpful in identifying the virus antigens. Immunostaining for p7, p9, p17, and p24 HIV protein recognizes the presence of the virus.

Castleman disease lymphadenopathy FNA cytologic samples do not allow one to make a specific diagnosis (Fig. 4.96); the presence of vascular capillary branching does not constitute a cytomorphologic hallmark. Immunocytochemistry may provide the diagnosis in the appropriate clinical context by highlighting HHV-8 antigens (Fig. 4.97), vascular structures (Fig. 4.98), and normal T- (Fig. 4.99) and B-lymphocyte populations (Fig. 4.100) with polyclonal kappa (Fig. 4.101) and lambda light chains (Fig. 4.102); or the absence of immunoglobulin gene rearrangement may be determined by molecular testing.

Sarcoidosis FNA cytology shows non-caseating granulomas composed of variable numbers of epithelioid histiocytes. The epithelioid histiocytes are oval, curved, or spindle-shaped; they have abundant cytoplasm with indistinct borders and curved or slightly indented nuclei. Necrosis is usually absent.

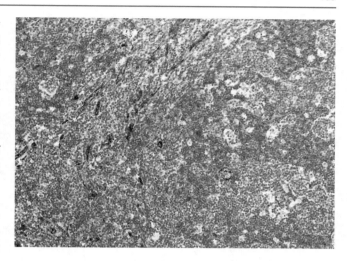

Fig. 4.98 Lymph node Castleman disease. CD34 immunostain (low magnification)

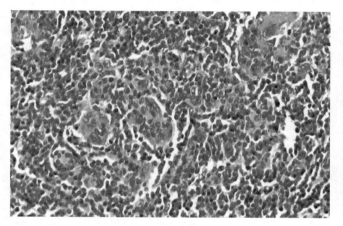

Fig. 4.96 Lymph node Castleman disease. Giemsa stain (high magnification)

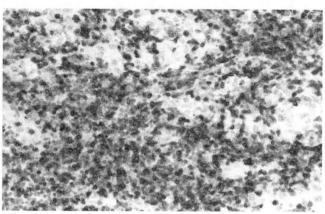

Fig. 4.99 Lymph node Castleman disease. CD3 immunostain (high magnification)

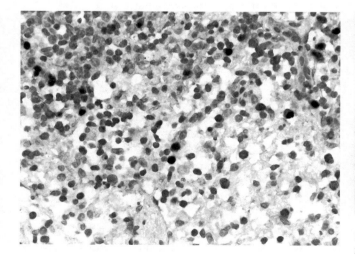

Fig. 4.97 Lymph node Castleman disease. HHV8 immunostain (high magnification)

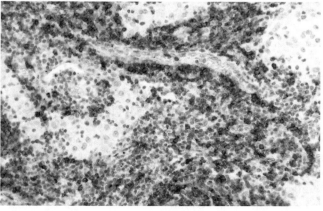

Fig. 4.100 Lymph node Castleman disease. CD20 immunostain (high magnification)

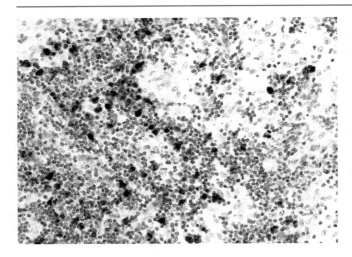

Fig. 4.101 Lymph node Castleman disease. Kappa light chains immunostain (high magnification)

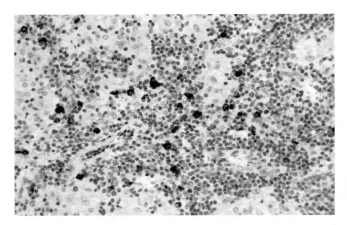

Fig. 4.102 Lymph node Castleman disease. Lambda light chains immunostain (high magnification)

Immunostainings with CD4, CD45, CD68, and S-100 protein give evidence for the histiocytic nature of the cells.

Rosai–Dorfman lymphadenopathy FNA cytology shows a mixture of small lymphocytes, plasmacytoid lymphocytes, immunoblasts, and histiocytes. If present in the cytologic preparations, the emperipolesis phenomenon is the cytomorphologic key to the diagnosis of this entity. The lymphocytes are immunoreactive with B- and T-cell markers without any specificity, whereas histiocytes are immunopositive for S-100 protein and CD68.

Langerhans cell histiocytosis FNA samples are characterized by cells with reniform or contorted nuclei without nucleoli; the cells are positive for CD1a, langerin, and S-100 protein. The cytologic samples usually show abundant eosinophils.

Kikuchi–Fujimoto lymphadenopathy FNA cytomorphology in the appropriate clinical setting allows us to diagnose this process as it is characterized by the presence of granular proteinaceous material and nuclear debris admixed with numerous lymphocytes, plasmacytoid monocytes (large cells with a moderate rim of cytoplasm and round, eccentrically placed nuclei with dense chromatin), immunoblasts, and histiocytes. Neutrophils are rare or absent. Histiocytes have abundant cytoplasm containing karyorrhectic debris and peripherally placed nuclei. CD123 and TCL-1 antibodies highlight plasmacytoid monocytes. Immunoblasts express CD30, whereas histiocytes are positive for lysozyme, myeloperoxidase, CD68, and CD163. T cells are predominantly CD8-positive, and some of them express cytotoxic molecules.

Dermatopathic lymphadenopathy FNA cytologic preparations show interdigitating dendritic cells, pigment-laden non-tingible-body macrophages, plasma cells, and lymphocytes. Interdigitating dendritic cells are positive for S-100 protein, fascin, CD4, and CD68, whereas macrophages are positive for CD68 and CD163. The lymphocytes are predominantly T cells that are positive for T-cell markers and consist mostly of CD4-positive cells with only a minor subset of CD8-positive cells. Molecular tests for T-cell receptor gene rearrangement are useful for eliminating lymph node involvement by mycosis fungoides or T-cell lymphoma.

4.5.4 Lymphomas

Morphologic evaluations of cytologic preparations of lymph nodes in clinically suspected lymphoproliferative disease are not sufficient for making a diagnosis of the specific type. The cytologic diagnosis needs to be supported by flow cytometry, immunocytochemistry, and molecular tests for determination of the clonality of lymphoid cells and for classifying the correct subtype of lymphoma.

Small-cell lymphocytic lymphoma Cytology smears show a monomorphic pattern of small lymphocytes with scant basophilic cytoplasm, round nuclei with coarse chromatin, and inconspicuous nucleoli. Some paraimmunoblasts can be observed. The neoplastic cells are positive for CD5, CD19, CD20, CD23, CD43, CD79a, bcl-2, and PAX-5. Also, they show a clonal restriction of light-chain immunoglobulin. CD38 and ZAP-70 are expressed in some cases. Trisomy 12, (13q14) deletion, t(11;14), and t(14;19) have been reported.

Marginal-zone lymphoma The cytologic samples are composed of small cells with a monocytoid appearance, centrocyte-like cells, and small- and medium-sized lymphocytes in various proportions. Plasma cell differentiation may be evident in some cases. The neoplastic cells show positivity for CD19, CD20, CD22, CD79a, and PAX-5. Trisomy 3 (60%) or t(11;18) is present in some cases.

Mantle cell lymphoma Cytologic preparations show monomorphic small- to intermediate-sized lymphoid cells with scant cytoplasm, nuclei with dispersed chromatin and irregular contours, and inconspicuous or small nucleoli. Rare lymphoplasmacytic cells, plasma cells, and histiocytes may be observed. Neoplastic cells express CD5, CD19, CD20, CD43, CD79a, PAX-5, FMC7, cyclin D1, SOX-11, and monoclonal immunoglobulin light-chain restriction. Almost all cases show a t(11;14)(q13;q32) translocation.

Follicular lymphoma Depending on the subtype of follicular lymphoma, different cytology FNA patterns are present. In the small-cell subtype, there is a monotonous proliferation of centrocytes with scant cytoplasm, irregular nuclei with notches, and nonparent nucleoli. The mixed cell subtype shows a mixture of centrocytes and centroblasts (large cells with relatively abundant basophilic cytoplasm and round nuclei with one to three nucleoli placed on the nuclear membrane). Sometimes, cell aggregates are present, suggesting a nodular lesion. Neoplastic cells are positive for CD10, CD19, CD20, CD79a, PAX-5, bcl-2, bcl-6, and immunoglobulin light-chain monoclonality. Almost all cases show a t(14;18) translocation.

Large-cell B-cell lymphoma (LCBCL) FNA cytologic preparations show large lymphoid cells which have variable cytomorphology and are composed of a mixture of centroblasts and immunoblasts, sometimes including large cells with irregular, multilobed nuclei. Neoplastic cells are positive for CD19, CD20, CD79a, PAX-5, and restricted light-chain immunoglobulin. The neoplastic cells of the GCB (germinal center B cells) subtype are immunoreactive for CD10 and bcl-6, whereas those of the ABC (activated B cells) variant show positivity for MUM-1/IRF4 and sometimes for bcl-6. Some cases show *c-myc* and *bcl-2* and/or *bcl-6* rearrangement (high-grade B-cell lymphoma double hit and triple hit). The anaplastic variant of LCBCL shows large and/or giant pleomorphic cells with abundant clear cytoplasm and irregular nuclei mimicking the pathognomonic cells of Hodgkin lymphoma. The neoplastic cells are positive for CD19, CD20, CD30, CD79a, and PAX-5. Some cells are also immunoreactive with bcl-6 and MUM-1/IRF4. The ALKoma variant expresses CD30, CD138, EMA, MUM-1/IRF4, and ALK.

Burkitt lymphoma FNA cytology shows medium-sized lymphoid cells with moderate, deeply basophilic, but some-

times vacuolated cytoplasm and round nuclei with evenly distributed chromatin and one or multiple prominent nucleoli (Fig. 4.103). Usually, numerous mitoses and apoptotic cells are seen in the background and are also present in the macrophage cytoplasm. Immunocytochemistry and flow cytometry substantiate the monoclonality of B cells, which are also positive for CD10 (Fig. 4.104), CD19, CD20 (Fig. 4.105), CD43, CD74, CD79a, PAX-5, and c-myc (Fig. 4.106). Antigens and DNA EBV (Fig. 4.107) are present in endemic Burkitt and in approximately 30% of sporadic and immunodeficiency-associated Burkitt lymphomas. Molecular testing detects t(8;14) (q24; q32), t(2;8)(p12; q24), or t(8;22) (q24; q11) translocations.

Lymphoblastic B-cell lymphoma FNA cytology shows small- to intermediate-sized lymphoid cells with scant cytoplasm, round or occasionally cleaved nuclei with fine and

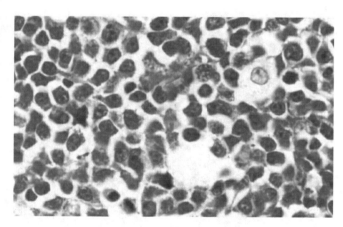

Fig. 4.103 Lymph node Burkitt lymphoma. Giemsa stain (high magnification)

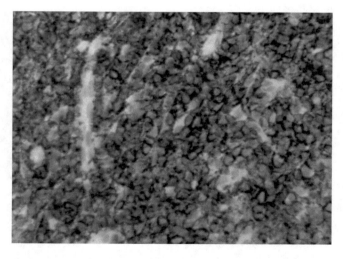

Fig. 4.104 Lymph node Burkitt lymphoma. CD10 immunostain (high magnification)

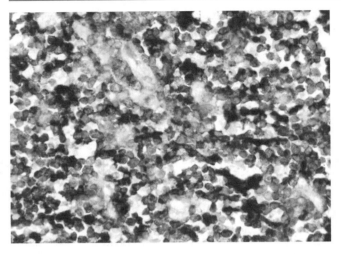

Fig. 4.105 Lymph node Burkitt lymphoma. CD20 immunostain (high magnification)

delicate chromatin, and variable presence of prominent nucleoli. The neoplastic cells are positive for terminal deoxynucleotidyl transferase (TdT), CD10, CD19, and PAX-5. CD20, CD22, CD24, and CD79a are usually expressed in the cytoplasm and not in the cytoplasmic membrane.

Lymphoblastic T-cell lymphoma Neoplastic cells are similar to those of the B-cell counterpart, even if intermediate-sized cells predominate. These cells show a moderate amount of cytoplasm, often irregular, cleaved nuclei, fine and delicate chromatin, and one to three small nucleoli (Fig. 4.108). The neoplastic cells usually show cytoplasmic CD3 (Fig. 4.109), CD7, and TdT (Fig. 4.110). Depending on their grade of "maturation," the neoplastic cells may display positivity for CD1a, CD2, CD4, CD5, CD8, CD10, CD34, and CD38. T-cell receptor gene rearrangements, commonly of α and δ loci, are usually present.

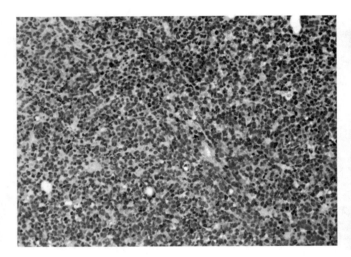

Fig. 4.106 Lymph node Burkitt lymphoma. c-myc immunostain (high magnification)

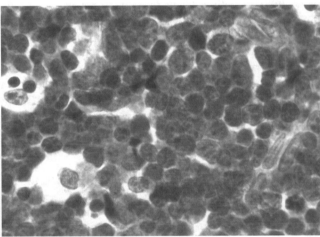

Fig. 4.108 Lymph node T-lymphoblastic lymphoma. Giemsa stain (high magnification)

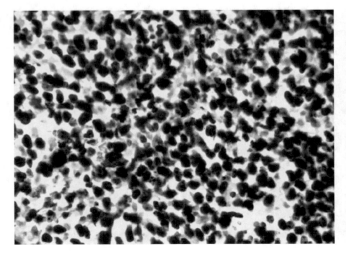

Fig. 4.107 Lymph node Burkitt lymphoma. EBER ISH (high magnification)

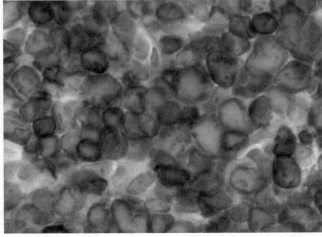

Fig. 4.109 Lymph node T-lymphoblastic lymphoma. CD3 immunostain (high magnification)

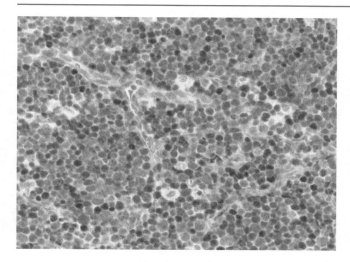

Fig. 4.110 Lymph node T-lymphoblastic lymphoma. TdT immunostain (high magnification)

Adult T-cell leukemia/lymphoma FNA cytologic preparations are characterized by neoplastic lymphoid cells of intermediate to large and sometimes giant size with relatively abundant clear cytoplasm, marked nuclear irregularities, coarse chromatin, and prominent nucleoli; convoluted nuclei may be observed. Tumor cells express CD2, CD3, CD5, CD25, CD29, CD30, CD38, CD71, CCR4, FOXP3, and HLA-DR. In most cases, CD4-positive cells and, in rare cases, CD8-positive cells are present. Rarely, co-expression of CD4 and CD8 on the same cell is observed. Viral antigens, such as p40 protein and HBZ, and viral nucleic acid may be detected by immunocytochemistry and molecular biology.

Peripheral T-cell lymphoma FNA cytologic samples usually show a polymorphous pattern consisting of various combinations of small, intermediate, and large cells, sometimes with Reed–Sternberg cell-like appearance. Neoplastic cells have a clear cytoplasm, irregular nuclei, and prominent nucleoli. This lymphoma exhibits a complicated immunophenotype: CD3 is usually expressed in the cell membrane; sometimes this molecule is present only in the cytoplasm, and in a few cases it may be detected only by flow cytometry because of its low density. Neoplastic cells are also positive for CD2, CD43, and CD45RO and, in most cases, for CD4 and CD30. Rare cases lack CD4 and express CD8. Most lymphomas express TCR α/β and present a rearranged TCR.

Sézary syndrome FNA cytology shows that the same cells found in the skin and in peripheral blood are affected by this process. The neoplastic cells (Sézary cells) have a small to intermediate size, moderate amounts of cytoplasm, and irregular "cerebriform" nuclei, sometimes with a monocytoid appearance, and one to three nucleoli. The neoplastic cells are immunoreactive with CD2, CD3, CD5, cutaneous lymphocyte antigen (CLA), the skin-homing receptor CCR4, and

TCRβ. Most cases are CD4-positive, and rare cases are CD8-positive. T-cell receptor gene rearrangement is present.

Anaplastic large-cell lymphoma FNA cytologic preparations show large or very large cells with abundant clear or basophilic cytoplasm, sometimes with small vacuoles and peripheral blebs, horseshoe- or kidney-shaped nuclei with prominent clear perinuclear hofs, and round or angular and prominent nucleoli. Neoplastic cells may appear as "doughnut cells," multinucleated giant "wreath cells," "embryo cells," "tennis-racket" or "hand mirror" cells, and cells with polylobate nuclei resembling Reed–Sternberg cells. Tumor cells usually express CD2, CD4, CD5, CD30 (with membrane and Golgi pattern), CD45, and EMA. Most cases are ALK-positive and present a t(2;5) or t(1;2) translocation.

Hodgkin lymphoma Cytologic samples show a background of reactive polymorphous lymphoid cells with predominance of small mature lymphocytes and variable numbers of eosinophils, plasma cells, and even epithelioid cells that sometimes simulate a granulomatous lymphadenitis. The diagnosis requires identification of the pathognomonic Reed–Sternberg and Hodgkin cells that usually have a moderate amount of pale cytoplasm with one or more eccentrically placed large, lobulated nuclei with irregular borders, coarse chromatin, and prominent irregular eosinophilic nucleoli (Fig. 4.111). The neoplastic cells show positivity for CD15 (Fig. 4.112), CD30 (Fig. 4.113), PAX-5, and BOB.1.

4.5.5 Lymph Node Metastases

FNA cytology of superficial lymph nodes is useful for verifying the presence of metastases in the case of known primary tumors. This practice is also useful for identifying a metastatic

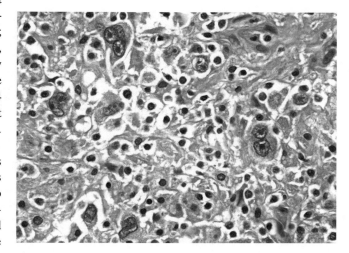

Fig. 4.111 Lymph node Hodgkin lymphoma. H&E stain (high magnification)

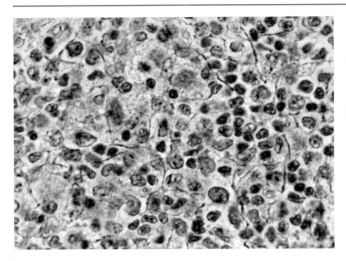

Fig. 4.112 Lymph node Hodgkin lymphoma. CD15 immunostain (high magnification)

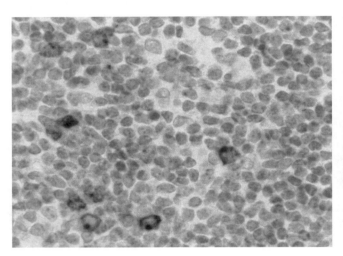

Fig. 4.113 Lymph node Hodgkin lymphoma. CD30 immunostain (high magnification)

deposit in patients who have an occult primary neoplasm. Common metastases include different variants of adenocarcinoma, squamous cell carcinoma, poorly differentiated small carcinoma, large-cell carcinoma, and melanoma. Less common lesions are thyroid carcinoma, nasopharyngeal carcinoma, urothelial carcinoma, germ cell tumors, and neuroendocrine tumors. Metastases of mesenchymal tumors such as Kaposi's sarcoma, Ewing sarcoma, rhabdomyosarcoma, synovial sarcoma, clear-cell sarcoma, epithelioid sarcoma, and angiosarcoma are rare. The clinical data and cytomorphology suggest the nature and origin of the metastatic deposit, and immunocytochemistry, molecular tests, and genetic properties may be used for refining and making the correct diagnosis.

Metastatic breast carcinoma FNA cytology of the ductal variant shows aggregates or slightly cohesive neoplastic cells

with pale cytoplasm and eccentrically placed nuclei (Fig. 4.114). In metastases of the lobular variant of breast adenocarcinoma, some tumor cells display intracytoplasmic vacuoles and eccentric nuclei. In the mucinous subtype, there is a mucinous background. Immunocytochemistry, independent of the subtype, is positive for CK7 and GATA-3 (Fig. 4.115) and variably positive for mammaglobin (Fig. 4.116) and GCFDP-15. Positive ER and PgR expression is seen in some cases.

Metastatic adenocarcinoma of the lung Cytologic preparations show slightly cohesive neoplastic cells with ample cytoplasm, some of which have intracytoplasmic vacuoles and round or irregular nuclei with prominent nucleoli. The neoplastic cells have positivity for CK7, TTF-1, and/or napsin A.

Metastatic gastric cancer FNA samples usually show small clusters and single neoplastic cells that have scanty, sometimes

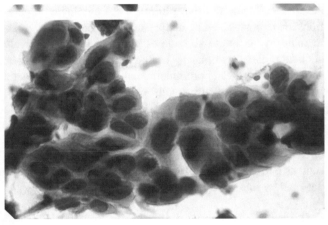

Fig. 4.114 Lymph node breast cancer metastasis. H&E stain (high magnification)

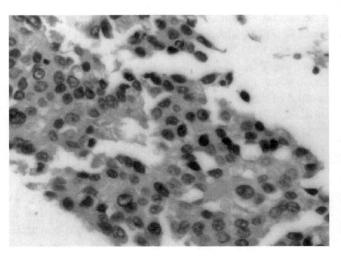

Fig. 4.115 Lymph node breast cancer metastasis. GATA-3 immunostain (high magnification)

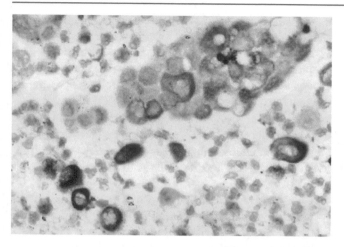

Fig. 4.116 Lymph node breast cancer metastasis. Mammaglobin immunostain (high magnification)

vacuolated cytoplasm with a signet-ring appearance and round or irregular nuclei usually with prominent nucleoli. Immunocytochemistry is positive for CK7 and/or CK20 or only for CK8 and CK18, HepPar antigen, CDX-2, and pS2 protein.

Metastatic colon carcinoma Lymph node FNA cytology shows groups of cohesive and large aggregates of cancer cells, sometimes with a cylindrical appearance. Neoplastic cells are positive for CK20 and CDX-2.

Metastatic ovarian serous papillary carcinoma Cytologic preparations show an acinar or papillary organization of the cancer cells, with a mesothelium-like appearance. Neoplastic cells have positivity for CK7, WT-1, PAX-8, CA125, EMA, and B72.3.

Metastatic squamous carcinoma When the carcinoma is well-differentiated, smears show high cellularity and exhibit keratinized cells, with hyperchromatic enlarged and sometimes pyknotic nuclei. Poorly differentiated squamous cell carcinoma shows cellular anaplasia, and the cytoplasm often lacks keratinization. Independent of cellular differentiation, immunocytochemistry is positive for CK5, desmocollin-3, p40, and sometimes p63.

Metastatic nasopharyngeal carcinoma Cytologic samples show aggregates of cells, sometimes with basaloid organization, and single cells with round or elongated features, scant cytoplasm, large nuclei, and prominent nucleoli. Lymphocytes, necrosis, and mitosis are commonly present. The neoplastic cells are positive for CK5, CK14, and p40 and occasionally for p63, desmoplakin 1-2, and EMA. Immunostains with EBV antigens such as LMP-1 and LMP-2 protein and in situ hybridization with encoded RNA (EBER) are useful.

Metastatic thyroid carcinoma Neoplastic cells may be highlighted by immunostainings with CK7, CK19, thyroglobulin, TTF-1, HBME-1, PAX-8, COX-2, and galectin-3. Cytology smears from the metastatic medullary subtype show dispersed small- to medium-sized cells with variable, usually ample cytoplasm, peripherally located round nuclei with fine chromatin, and small, inconspicuous nucleoli. Neoplastic cells immunoreact with low-molecular-weight CK (except CK7), calcitonin, chromogranin A, synaptophysin, NSE, CEA, CD56, and CD57. Cells express calcitonin-related peptide and somatostatin.

Metastatic melanoma The diagnosis is relatively easy if the clinical history is known and if FNA cytology shows neoplastic cells containing melanin pigment. Cytologic samples are usually cellular and are composed of oval, round, or spindle-shaped cells with pleomorphic nuclei, sometimes with nuclear pseudoinclusions, and prominent nucleoli (Figs. 4.117 and 4.118). In case of metastases from amelanotic melanoma, the cytomorphology may suggest the diagnosis and it should be confirmed by use of immunostains, such as S-100 protein, melan-A (Fig. 4.119), HMB-45 (Fig. 4.120), and SOX-10.

Metastatic neuroendocrine carcinoma Cytologic preparations are composed of small- to intermediate-sized, usually non-cohesive neoplastic cells with scant cytoplasm, round nuclei with fine chromatin, and small nucleoli. The neoplastic cells are positive for CK8, CK18, CK19, NSE, chromogranin A, and synaptophysin. Metastases from *Merkel cell carcinoma* express CK20 in addition to the previous markers.

Metastatic carcinomas from an unknown primary site These tumors represent about 1–5% of lymph node

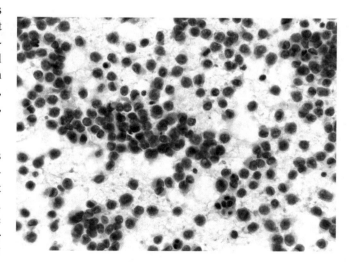

Fig. 4.117 Lymph node melanoma metastasis. Papanicolaou stain (high magnification)

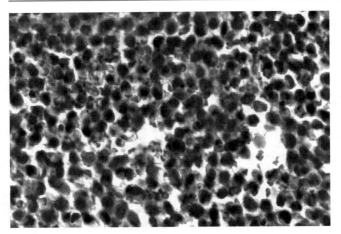

Fig. 4.118 Lymph node melanoma metastasis. H&E stain (high magnification)

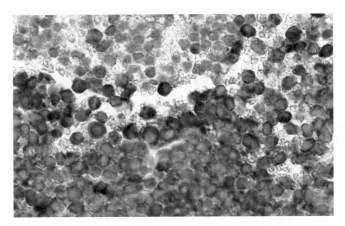

Fig. 4.119 Lymph node melanoma metastasis. Melan A immunostain (high magnification)

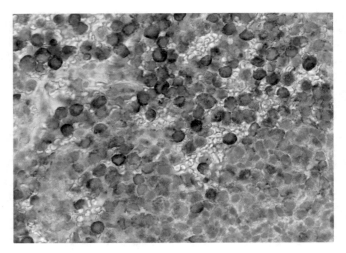

Fig. 4.120 Lymph node melanoma metastasis. HMB-45 immunostain (high magnification)

metastases. Patients have no obviously identifiable primary site, despite a careful clinical history, physical examination, imaging studies, and biochemical or invasive investigations. Cytomorphologically, the prevalent features are those of adenocarcinoma (about half of cases), followed by poorly differentiated carcinoma and neuroendocrine tumors.

It is useful to start the diagnostic approach by using CK7 and CK20 immunostaining, because the various stain results will narrow the diagnostic venues as follows:

1. CK7-positive and CK20-negative neoplastic cells are found in adenocarcinomas of the breast, lung, endometrium, ovary (serous, endometrioid, and clear cell), esophagus, thyroid, uterine cervix, kidney (papillary, chromophobe, and Bellini's ductal carcinoma), and salivary gland.
2. CK7-negative and CK20-positive neoplastic cells are observed in intestinal carcinoma and in about one third of gastric cancers.
3. CK7-negative and CK20-negative immunophenotype is present in neuroendocrine tumors (except Merkel carcinoma), squamous cell, prostate, hepatocellular (except the lamellar subtype), renal cell classic, adrenal gland, and about 10% of gastric carcinomas.
4. CK7-positive and CK20-positive immunophenotype characterizes neoplastic cells of exocrine pancreas, urothelial, mucinous ovarian, gallbladder, and some gastric carcinomas.

Subsequent markers must be applied for determination of the diagnosis as shown in Tables 4.1, 4.2, 4.3, and 4.4.

Table 4.1 Further markers for CK7-positive CK20-negative neoplastic cells

Markers	Diagnosis
TTF-1, napsin A	Lung adenocarcinoma
GATA-3, GCDFP-15, mammaglobin	Breast cancer
Vimentin, PAX-2	Endometrial cancer
WT-1, PAX-2	Serous and endometrioid ovarian cancer
Thyroglobulin, PAX-8	Papillary and follicular thyroid cancer
Calcitonin, chromogranin A, CEA	Medullary thyroid cancer
p16	Uterine cervix cancer
Cyclin D1	Esophagus cancer
RCC, PAX-8	Renal cell carcinoma (except clear cell)
p63, S-100 protein	Salivary gland carcinoma
pS2, HepPar	Gastric cancer
HepPar	Hepatocellular carcinoma, lamellar subtype

Table 4.2 Further markers for CK7-positive, CK20-positive neoplastic cells

Markers	Diagnosis
CDX-2	Large bowel carcinoma
SIMA	Small bowel carcinoma
pS2, HepPar	Gastric adenocarcinoma
Chromogranin A, CD56	Merkel cell carcinoma

Table 4.3 Further markers for CK7-negative, CK20-negative neoplastic cells

Markers	Diagnosis
p63, p40, desmollin-3	Squamous cell carcinoma
PSA, PSMA, AMACR	Prostate carcinoma
HepPar, TTF-1 (cytoplasm)	Hepatocellular carcinoma (except lamellar)
Chromogranin A, synaptophysin, CD56	Neuroendocrine carcinoma
Melan A, inhibin-α	Adrenal gland carcinoma
pS2, HepPar	Gastric carcinoma
RCC, PAX-2, CD10	Renal cell clear-cell carcinoma
Lipase, trypsin	Acinic cell exocrine pancreatic carcinoma

Table 4.4 Further markers for CK7-positive, CK20-positive neoplastic cells

Markers	Diagnosis
CK17, DUPAN-2	Ductal cell exocrine pancreatic carcinoma
GATA-3, p63, thrombomodulin, uroplakin III	Urothelial carcinoma
HAM56	Ovarian mucinous carcinoma
pS2, HepPar	Gastric carcinoma

Suggested Reading

Agarwal A, et al. Parathyroid fine-needle aspiration cytology in the evaluation of parathyroid adenoma: Cytologic findings from 53 patients. Diagn Cytopathol. 2009;37:407.

Bardales RH. The invasive cytopathologist. Ultrasound guided fine-needle aspiration of superficial masses. New York: Springer; 2014.

Cha H, et al. The usefulness of immunocytochemistry of CD56 in determining malignancy from indeterminate thyroid fine-needle aspiration cytology. J Pathol Transl Med. 2018;52:404.

Fischer S, Asa SL. Application of immunohistochemistry to thyroid neoplasms. Arch Pathol Lab Med. 2008;132:359.

Frederiksen JK, et al. Systematic review of the effectiveness of fine-needle aspiration and/or core needle biopsy for subclassifying lymphoma. Arch Pathol Lab Med. 2015;139:245.

Gherardi G. Fine-needle biopsy of superficial and deep masses. Milano: Springer; 2009.

Kazi M, et al. Fine-needle aspiration cytology (FNAC) in breast cancer: a reappraisal based on retrospective review of 698 cases. World J Surg. 2017;41:1528.

Kocjan G, et al. BSCC code of practice – fine needle aspiration cytology. Cytopathology. 2009;20:283.

Mehanna HM, et al. Investigating the thyroid nodule. BMJ. 2009;338:b733.

Schmidt RL, et al. A systematic review and meta-analysis of the diagnostic accuracy of fine-needle aspiration cytology for parotid gland lesions. Am J Clin Pathol. 2011;136:45.

Sergi C, et al. Fine needle aspiration cytology for neck masses in childhood. An illustrative approach. Diagnostics. 2018;8:28.

Tracy TF Jr, Muratore CS. Management of common head and neck masses. Semin Pediatr Surg. 2007;16:3.

Fine-needle aspiration (FNA) cytology is a minimally inva-sive procedure that allows obtaining material from deep-seated masses for a rapid and accurate diagnosis. Cytomorphologic analysis determines the correct nature of the lesion and provides a conclusion whether the mass is neoplastic (benign or malignant) or non-neoplastic. Immunocytochemistry is a paramount means for refining the morphologic diagnosis and guiding further clinical manage-ment of the patient.

5.1 Lung Masses

Cytologic samples of peripheral lung masses, which are not easy to harvest via an endobronchial approach, may be obtained by percutaneous transthoracic FNA with the use of computed tomography (CT), fluoroscopy, ultrasound (US), or magnetic resonance imaging guidance. Usually, FNA samples are suitable for smear preparations, cell block, and ancillary tests, i.e., cultures, immunocytochemistry, molecu-lar or genetic studies, flow cytometry, and electron micros-copy, as clinically appropriate.

5.1.1 Lung Adenocarcinoma

In a well-differentiated adenocarcinoma, smears and cell-block cytology show tissue fragments, some with luminal spaces lined by tall columnar cells with oval nuclei, a bland chromatin pattern, and small nucleoli. In some cases, there are single-cell layers with architectural abnormalities, nuclei of different sizes, and a variable nuclear-to-cytoplasmic ratio. Moderately differentiated lung adenocarcinomas pre-dominantly show tissue fragments with an evident glandular pattern or sometimes with papillary features. Neoplastic cells show fair amounts of cytoplasm with distinct borders and, sometimes, with secretory vacuoles and round to oval nuclei with prominent nucleoli. Cytologic preparations from

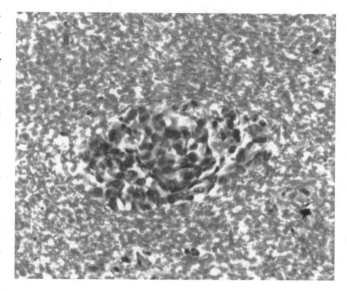

Fig. 5.1 Lung adenocarcinoma. H&E (high magnification)

poorly differentiated adenocarcinoma are composed of neo-plastic cells with rare secretory vacuoles, pleomorphic nuclei, and prominent nucleoli; cells are predominantly arranged in complex tissue fragments (Fig. 5.1). Independent of the grade of differentiation, neoplastic cells are positive for CK7 (Fig. 5.2), TTF-1 (Fig. 5.3), and/or napsin A, EMA, CEA, ERA, ESA, and B72.3. The mucinous subtype expresses CK7 and CK20, but it is TTF-1-negative.

5.1.2 Metastases to the Lung

The occurrence of multiple lung nodules favors the presence of a metastatic deposit, mainly adenocarcinoma, although primary tumors may occasionally be multicentric. Correlation with clinical data, including imaging studies, cytomorphol-ogy, and ancillary tests, is necessary for determining the pos-

© Springer Nature Switzerland AG 2020
E. Leonardo, R. H. Bardales, *Practical Immunocytochemistry in Diagnostic Cytology*,
https://doi.org/10.1007/978-3-030-46656-5_5

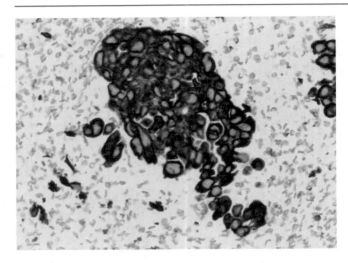

Fig. 5.2 Lung adenocarcinoma. CK7 immunostain (high magnification)

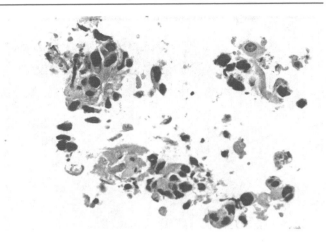

Fig. 5.4 Colon cancer metastatic cells. H&E (high magnification)

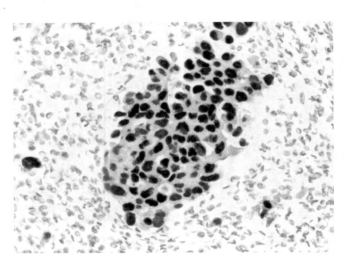

Fig. 5.3 Lung adenocarcinoma. TTF-1 immunostain (high magnification)

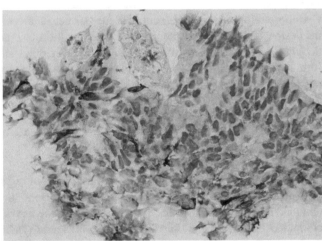

Fig. 5.5 Colon cancer metastatic cells. CK20 immunostain (high magnification)

sible source of a metastasis. The use of formalin-fixed, paraffin-embedded cell-block material is always preferable to the performance of ancillary tests, including immunohistochemistry. Morphologically, the cytologic features of the FNA samples may be grouped in various patterns for construction of a differential diagnosis.

Acinar/glandular pattern This architecture usually is related to colorectal (Fig. 5.4), pancreatobiliary, or prostatic adenocarcinoma. Neoplastic cells of colonic carcinoma express CK20 (Fig. 5.5) and CDX-2 (Fig. 5.6); cells of pancreatobiliary carcinoma express CK8, CK18, and variable amounts of CK20, DUPAN-2, E-cadherin protein, and claudin 7; prostate neoplastic cells are positive for PSA, PSMA, and AMACR.

Signet-ring cell pattern Metastatic adenocarcinoma with a signet-ring-cell/mucinous pattern originates from the breast (Fig. 5.7), ovary (Fig. 5.8), or digestive system – mainly the stomach (Fig. 5.9). Breast carcinoma cells immunoreact with CK7 and GATA-3 (Fig. 5.10) and, in variable amounts, with mammaglobin and GCFDP-15. Colorectal carcinoma is immunopositive for CK20, CDX-2, and nuclear β-catenin, whereas gastric cancer expresses HepPar, pS2, MUC-6, and, in variable proportions, CK7 and CK20. Neoplastic cells of mucinous ovarian cancers are positive for CK7, WT-1, PAX-8, and CA125, and some cells for CK20.

Papillary pattern The differential diagnosis includes serous ovarian carcinoma (Fig. 5.11), serous endometrial cancer, thyroid carcinoma, renal cell carcinoma, mesothelioma, and colorectal cancer. Neoplastic cells of serous ovarian carcinoma express CK7, WT-1 (Fig. 5.12), PAX-8, and

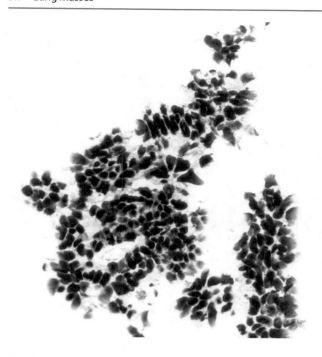

Fig. 5.6 Colon cancer metastatic cells. CDX-2 immunostain (high magnification)

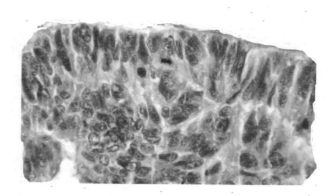

Fig. 5.8 Mucinous ovary cancer metastatic cells. H&E (high magnification)

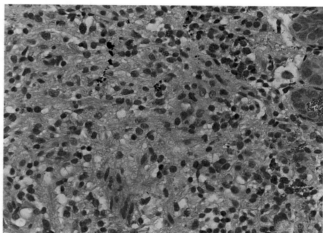

Fig. 5.9 Gastric cancer metastatic cells. H&E (high magnification)

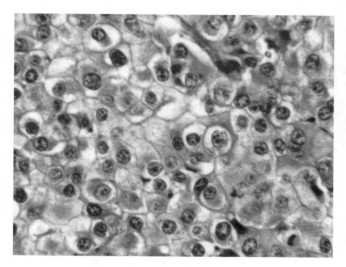

Fig. 5.7 Breast cancer metastatic cells. H&E (high magnification)

B72.3. Tumor cells of serous endometrial cancer are immunoreactive with CK7, PAX-8, and cytoplasmic β-catenin, and some cells immunoreactive with WT-1. CK7, CK19, thyroglobulin, HBME-1, galectin-3, and PAX-8 are present in metastases of thyroid carcinoma. Metastatic cells of papillary renal cell carcinoma (Fig. 5.13) show positivity for CK7 (Fig. 5.14), PAX-2, and RCC. Neoplastic mesothelial cells (Fig. 5.15) are immunopositive for CK5, WT-1, calretinin (Fig. 5.16), and podoplanin. Colorectal metastatic cells have an immunophenotype characterized by positivity for CK20, CDX-2, and nuclear β-catenin.

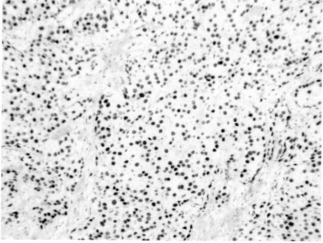

Fig. 5.10 Breast cancer metastatic cells GATA-3 immunostain (high magnification)

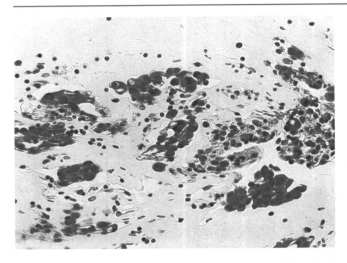

Fig. 5.11 Serous ovary cancer metastatic cells. H&E (high magnification)

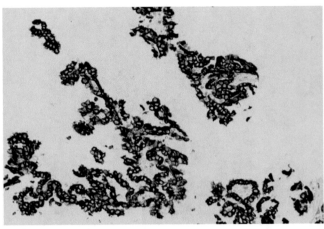

Fig. 5.14 Papillary renal cancer metastatic cells. CK7 immunostain (high magnification)

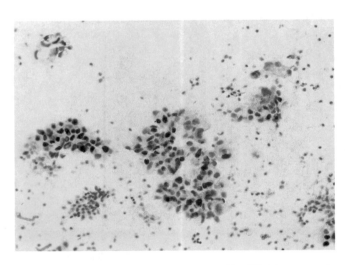

Fig. 5.12 Serous ovary cancer metastatic cells. WT-1 immunostain (high magnification)

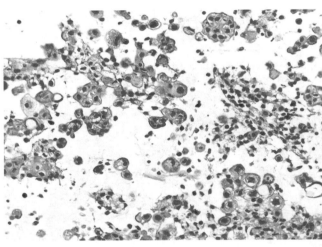

Fig. 5.15 Mesothelioma metastatic cells H&E (high magnification)

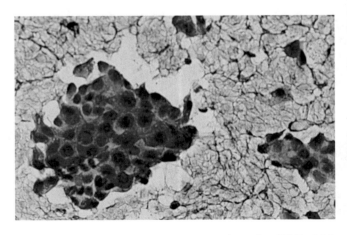

Fig. 5.13 Papillary renal cancer metastatic cells. H&E (high magnification)

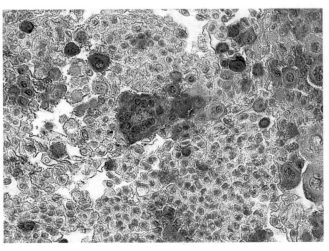

Fig. 5.16 Mesothelioma metastatic cells. Calretinin immunostain (high magnification)

Solid nest pattern Metastatic carcinomas with this pattern mainly include breast adenocarcinoma, squamous cell carcinoma, hepatocellular carcinoma, and urothelial carcinoma. Neoplastic breast cancer cells express CK7 and GATA-3; some cells are also positive for mammaglobin and GCFDP-15. Squamous cell carcinoma metastasis (usually from head and neck cancer) is indistinguishable from primary or metastatic squamous cell lung cancer, because the cells express the same immunophenotype, i.e., positivity for CK5 (Fig. 5.17), p40 protein (Fig. 5.18), and desmocollin-3. Metastatic tumors originating in the cervix are positive for CK5 and p16 protein, indicating the high-risk HPV involvement. Immunocytochemistry in metastatic hepatocellular carcinoma (Fig. 5.19) exhibits positivity for CK8, CK18, HepPar (Fig. 5.20), and glyplican-3. Metastatic urothelial carcinoma cells immunoreact with CK7, GATA-3 (Fig. 5.21), and p63 protein (Fig. 5.22) and sometimes with CK20.

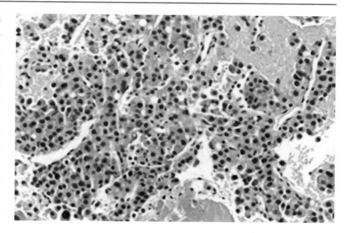

Fig. 5.19 Hepatocellular carcinoma metastatic cells. H&E (high magnification)

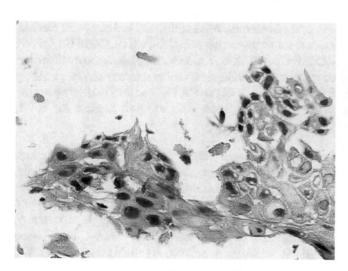

Fig. 5.17 Squamous cell carcinoma metastatic cells. H&E (high magnification)

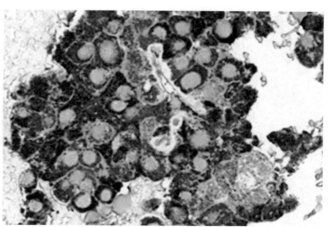

Fig. 5.20 Hepatocellular carcinoma metastatic cells. HepPar immunostain (high magnification)

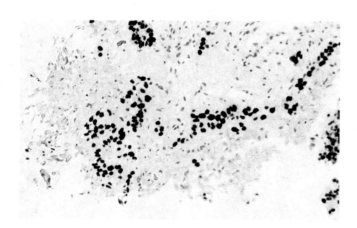

Fig. 5.18 Squamous cell carcinoma metastatic cells. p40 immunostain (high magnification)

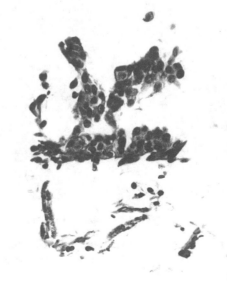

Fig. 5.21 Urothelial carcinoma metastatic cells. H&E (high magnification)

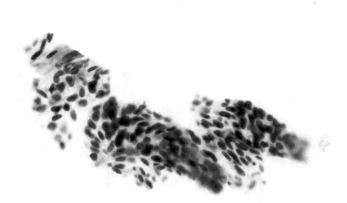

Fig. 5.22 Urothelial carcinoma metastatic cells. p63 immunostain (high magnification)

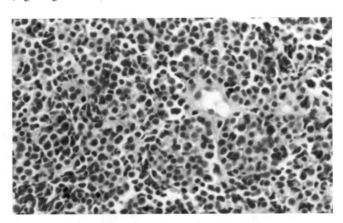

Fig. 5.23 Neuroendocrine carcinoma metastatic cells. H&E (high magnification)

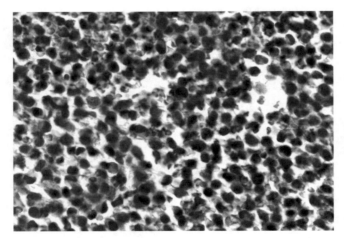

Fig. 5.24 Melanoma metastatic cells. H&E (high magnification)

Diffuse single-cell pattern This pattern is commonly seen in metastatic breast carcinoma, neuroendocrine carcinoma (Fig. 5.23), and melanoma (Fig. 5.24). Breast neoplastic cells have the immunophenotype reported in the solid nest pattern. Immunocytochemistry positive for CK8, CK18,

CK19, chromogranin A, synaptophysin, and CD56 is observed in neuroendocrine tumors. The presence of TTF-1 suggests a diagnosis of primary neuroendocrine lung cancer, whereas metastatic neuroendocrine cells positive for PDX-1 and CDX-2 usually originate in the stomach. Metastatic pancreatic neuroendocrine carcinomas express NESP55 and ISLET-1, and some express PDX-1. CDX-2, with some cells positive for PDX-1, is observed in metastatic neuroendocrine carcinoma from the cecal appendix, whereas neuroendocrine metastatic cells of the ileum express only CDX-2. Metastatic duodenal neuroendocrine carcinoma is positive for PDX-1. The diagnosis of metastatic melanoma is straightforward when single neoplastic cells or small clusters contain melanin pigment. In amelanotic melanoma, immunocytochemistry helps identify the positivity of neoplastic cells for S-100 protein, melan A, HMB-45, and SOX-10.

Clear-cell pattern Metastases showing this pattern include renal cell clear-cell carcinoma (Fig. 5.25) and ovarian clear-cell adenocarcinoma. Metastatic renal cell clear-cell carcinomas are immunoreactive with CK8, CK18, CD10 (Fig. 5.26), RCC, PAX-2, PAX-8, and vimentin. Immunocytochemistry of metastatic ovarian clear-cell carcinoma shows positivity for CK7, CK8, CK18, CK19, and HNF-1β (hepatocyte nuclear factor-1β); some cells are also positive for WT-1, OCT-4, and CD15.

Spindle cell pattern Metastases with this pattern include sarcomatoid carcinoma, melanoma, and mesothelioma. Metastatic sarcomatoid carcinoma expresses pan cytokeratin, vimentin, and sometimes EMA. Spindle cell metastatic melanoma is variably positive for S-100 protein, melan A, HMB-45, SOX-10, MAGE-1, Mel-CAM, and MITF. Metastatic mesothelioma is variably positive for CK5, WT-1, podoplanin, and calretinin.

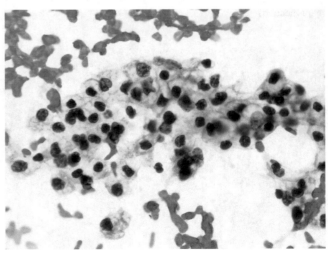

Fig. 5.25 Clear-cell renal cell metastatic cells. Papanicolaou (high magnification)

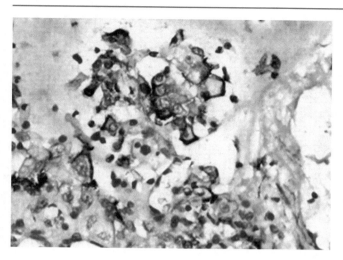

Fig. 5.26 Clear-cell renal cell metastatic cells. CD10 immunostain (high magnification)

Pleomorphic cell pattern Metastatic germ-cell tumors such as choriocarcinoma, embryonal carcinoma, and yolk sac tumors can originate in the ovary, testis, or mediastinum and occasionally involve the lung. Choriocarcinoma shows positivity for CK8, CK18, CK19, SALL-4, OCT-4, and PLAP; syncytiotrophoblasts, if present, express β-HCG. The immunocytochemistry of embryonal carcinoma is positive for CK8, CK18, CK19, SALL-4, OCT-4, PLAP, and CD30. Metastatic yolk sac tumors are immunoreactive for CK8, CK18, CK19, SALL-4, glypican-3, α-fetoprotein, and PLAP.

Non-epithelial cell pattern Metastatic tumors include different types of sarcomas, mainly leiomyosarcoma, endometrial stromal sarcoma, undifferentiated pleomorphic sarcoma, angiosarcoma, and synovial sarcoma. The neoplastic cells of *leiomyosarcoma* are immunopositive for vimentin, desmin, α-SMA, smooth muscle myosin, HHF-35, and h-caldesmon; some cells of the epithelioid variant may also express CK8, CK18, and S-100 protein. In *endometrial stromal sarcoma*, metastatic cells are positive for vimentin, CD10, and PgR and sometimes for ER and bcl-2. Metastatic *undifferentiated stromal sarcoma* is positive only for vimentin; some cells positive for CD68, CD10, CD99, and CD117 may be observed. Metastatic *angiosarcoma* shows positivity for CD31, CD34, CD105, FLI-1, and ERG, whereas F8Rag is occasionally present; the epithelioid angiosarcoma variant may express CK8. Metastatic *synovial sarcoma* usually shows positivity for vimentin, di CD99, bcl-2, TLE1, and SYT; some cells may immunoreact with calretinin, CK7, CK14, CK19, and EMA. Molecular biology helps one to identify the translocation t(X;18) (p11;q11).

5.2 Mediastinal Masses

FNA under radiologic (ultrasound, CT, etc.) guidance is a minimally invasive practice, is relatively economical, and is associated with a low risk of complications. Thus, this sampling modality has become the diagnostic strategy of choice for mediastinal masses.

5.2.1 Thymoma

Cytologic samples show variable cellularity and epithelial cells of varied cytomorphology, depending on the subtype of thymoma. Lymphocytes admixed with epithelial cells, which may be single or in small aggregates, tightly or loosely cohesive and round to polygonal or even spindle-shaped, may be observed. Epithelial cells of *type A thymoma* (Fig. 5.27) express CK13, CK14, CK15, CK16, CK17, CK18, and CK19, whereas the lymphocyte population is positive for CD3 (Fig. 5.28), CD4 or CD8, and CD5. Only a few lymphocytes are CD20-positive. Some epithelial cells may express CD20 and CD57. In *B1 thymoma subtype*, the epithelial cells are positive for CK19, and scattered elements also for CK7, CK14, CK15, and CK18. Lymphocytes exhibit an immature as well as a mature immunophenotype: the immature cells are immunoreactive with CD1a, with co-expression of CD4 and CD8, CD5, CD99, and TdT, whereas the mature lymphocytes are positive for CD2, CD3, CD5, and CD4 or CD8. The *B2 thymoma subtype* (Fig. 5.29) is characterized by positivity of epithelial cells for CK5 (Fig. 5.30), CK6, CK7, CK8, CK18, and CK19. The admixed lymphocytes are

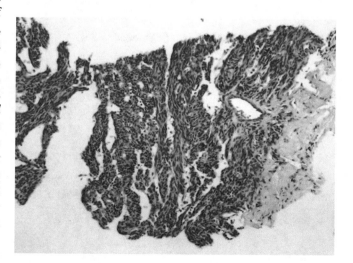

Fig. 5.27 Thymoma type A. H&E (high magnification)

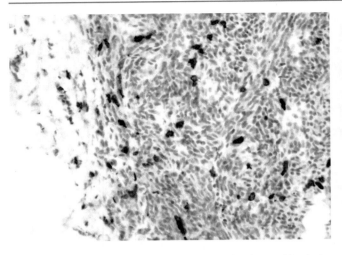

Fig. 5.28 Thymoma type A. CD3 immunostain (high magnification)

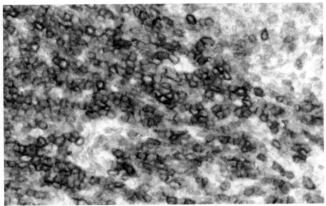

Fig. 5.31 Thymoma type B2. CD99 immunostain (high magnification)

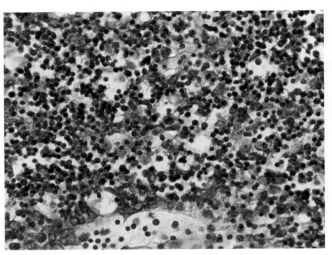

Fig. 5.29 Thymoma type B2. H&E (high magnification)

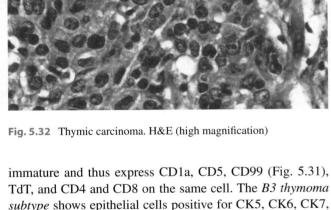

Fig. 5.32 Thymic carcinoma. H&E (high magnification)

immature and thus express CD1a, CD5, CD99 (Fig. 5.31), TdT, and CD4 and CD8 on the same cell. The *B3 thymoma subtype* shows epithelial cells positive for CK5, CK6, CK7, CK8, EMA, and CD57. The rare lymphocytes that are present have positivity for CD1a and CD4 and CD8 on the same cell, as well as CD5, CD99, and TdT.

5.2.2　Thymic Carcinoma

This neoplasia has a cytomorphologic pattern of poorly differentiated squamous cell carcinoma (Fig. 5.32). The neoplastic cells are immunoreactive for CK5, CK6, CK18, p63, p40 (Fig. 5.33), CD5 (Fig. 5.34), CD70, CD117, and GLUT-1. Some cells may also express CK8, CK13, CK16, and CK19.

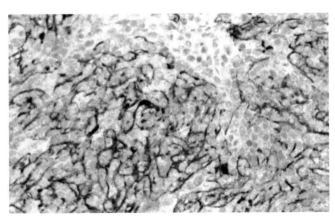

Fig. 5.30 Thymoma type B2. CK5 immunostain (high magnification)

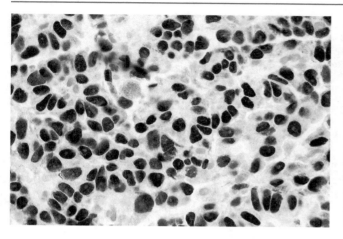

Fig. 5.33 Thymic carcinoma. p40 immunostain (high magnification)

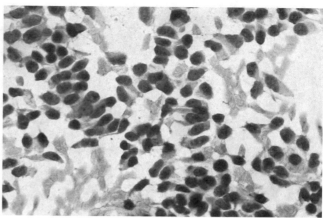

Fig. 5.35 Thymic carcinoid. H&E (high magnification)

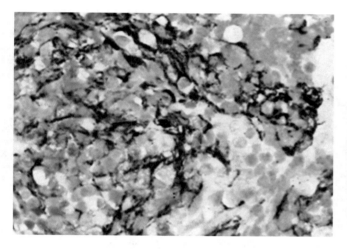

Fig. 5.34 Thymic carcinoma. CD5 immunostain (high magnification)

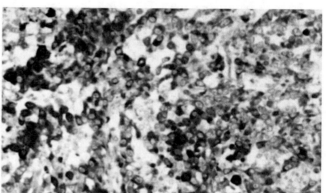

Fig. 5.36 Thymic carcinoid. Synaptophysin immunostain (high magnification)

5.2.3 Neuroendocrine Tumors

Thymic carcinoid The *typical thymic carcinoid variant* is usually composed of spindle-shaped or polygonal cells (Fig. 5.35), which express CK8, CK18, chromogranin A, synaptophysin (Fig. 5.36), CD56, and somatostatin receptors, mainly sst2A-R. Some cells may express CK20 and neuropeptides, such as ACTH, α-HCG, β-HCG, β-endorphin, neurotensin, and calcitonin. The *atypical thymic carcinoid variant* is also positive for CK19.

Neuroendocrine thymic carcinoma (Fig. 5.37) This tumor shows a pattern similar to that of neuroendocrine tumors at other anatomic sites. It expresses CK8, CK18, CK19, neuroendocrine markers (Fig. 5.38), and, in some cells, nuclear PAX-5 and CD99. The absence of TTF-1 allows differentiating this tumor from metastatic lung neuroendocrine carcinoma.

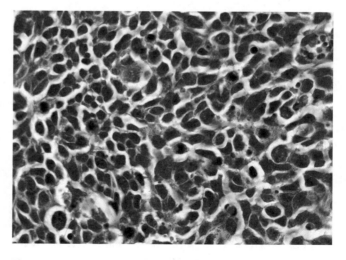

Fig. 5.37 Thymic neuroendocrine carcinoma, H&E (high magnification)

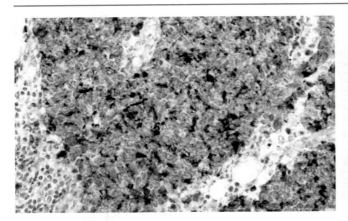

Fig. 5.38 Thymic neuroendocrine carcinoma, chromogranin A immunostain (high magnification)

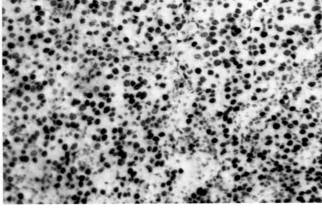

Fig. 5.40 Dysgerminoma. SALL-4 immunostain (high magnification)

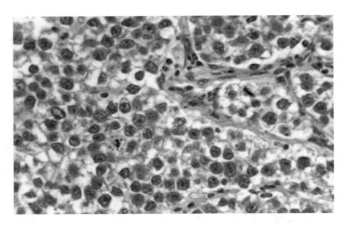

Fig. 5.39 Dysgerminoma. H&E (high magnification)

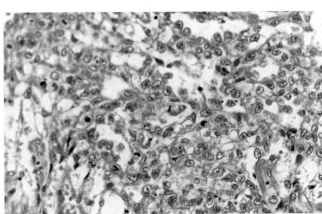

Fig. 5.41 Embryonal carcinoma. H&E (high magnification)

5.2.4　Germ-Cell Tumors

Seminoma and dysgerminoma Cytology samples show cells with clear or weakly eosinophilic cytoplasm (rich in glycogen) and a round nucleus with one or more prominent nucleoli (Fig. 5.39). Immunocytochemistry is positive for vimentin, SALL-4 (Fig. 5.40), OCT-4, PLAP, CD117, and OCT-4 (membrane or Golgian pattern). Low-molecular-weight cytokeratins (CK8 and CK18) can be expressed focally, with a low-intensity paranuclear pattern. Immunostaining for β-HCG highlights syncytiotrophoblastic elements when they present.

Embryonal carcinoma The cytology pattern shows large cells with an epithelial appearance and clear or granular cytoplasm; these cells aggregate to form solid, papillary, or glandular structures (Fig. 5.41). A particular marker of this neoplasm is CD30 (Fig. 5.42), which stains the cell membrane and sometimes the cytoplasm. The neoplastic cells are usually positive for SALL-4, OCT-4, CK7, CK8, CK18, and CK19, whereas positivity for α-fetoprotein and PLAP is

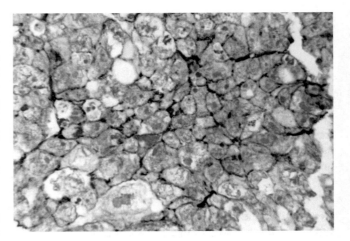

Fig. 5.42 Embryonal carcinoma. CD30 immunostain (high magnification)

observed only focally, in isolated tumor cells or in small group of cells. The possible presence of syncytiotrophoblastic elements would be highlighted by marking for β-HCG.

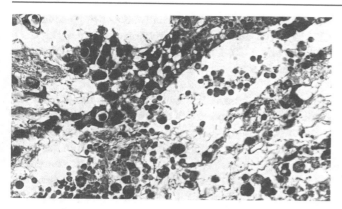

Fig. 5.43 Yolk sac tumor. H&E (high magnification)

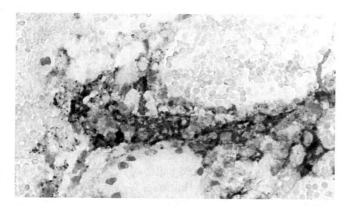

Fig. 5.44 Yolk sac tumor. Glyplican-3 immunostain (high magnification)

Yolk sac tumor The neoplastic cells are small and have round nuclei with small nucleoli that form small aggregates of glandular, alveolar, papillary, or solid-type configuration (Fig. 5.43). The neoplasm shows positivity for CK8, CK18, CK19, OCT-4, glyplican-3 (Fig. 5.44), and α-fetoprotein. Foci of neoplastic elements can show immunoreactivity for vimentin and CK7.

Choriocarcinoma Syncytiotrophoblasts can be detected by immunostaining for SALL-4, OCT-4, β-HCG, CK7, CK8, CK18, and CK19. Low-molecular-weight cytokeratins (LMW-CK) are distributed variably in the cytotrophoblast elements, which are also positive for human placental lactogen. Intermediate-type trophoblastic cells have LMW-CK as markers.

5.2.5 Mediastinal Lymphadenopathy

Endoscopy ultrasound (EUS) can easily identify lymph nodes of the sub-carinal, paraesophageal, and paratracheal regions, but not those of the pretracheal space or of intrapulmonary regions. Therefore, the combined use of EUS with fine-needle aspiration (EUS-FNA) allows sampling of the lymph nodes from these anatomic areas that may be suspected to harbor benign or malignant pathologic findings.

Infectious lymphadenopathy This is one of the most frequent causes of adenopathy as sampled by EUS-FNA. Mycobacteriosis and histoplasmosis are the most common infectious pathologies in mediastinal lymphadenopathy. Cytologic preparations show lymphocytes, granulomas, and necrosis in various proportions. Clinical-epidemiologic correlations are useful together with dedicated histochemical staining while molecular test results are pending. Immunocytochemical investigations do not offer any useful support for a diagnosis, because negative immunostaining does not exclude an infectious process nor confirm the presence of a noninfectious inflammatory lesion.

The presence of amorphous granular material and crystals, in the absence of granulomas in FNA cytologic samples, does not exclude a fungal infection; indeed, these findings are frequently observed in histoplasmosis.

The finding of granulomas, lymphocytes, and necrosis, associated with large capsulated yeast-like elements, is often observed in cryptococcal lymphadenitis, which is seen frequently in immunosuppressed subjects.

In sarcoidosis, cytologic preparations usually show poor cellularity, cohesive epithelioid granulomas, cellular degeneration, and often absence of necrosis. Negative findings on microbiological investigations and on clinical-radiologic studies are paramount for making the correct diagnosis.

Non-Hodgkin lymphoma This neoplasm can involve the thymus and/or mediastinal lymph nodes, either as a primary lesion or as a part of disseminated disease. At the thymic level, lymphomas frequently are marginal-zone B-cell lymphomas, primary mediastinal large B-cell lymphomas with sclerosis, lymphoblastic lymphomas, anaplastic lymphomas, or Hodgkin lymphomas, whereas in the mediastinal lymph nodes, any subtype of lymphoproliferative disease can develop. FNA cytology of *marginal-zone B-cell lymphoma* shows the same features observed in others organs: a mixed population of marginal-zone B-lymphocytes or monocytoid B cells, lymphoplasmacytes, plasmacytoid cells, scattered immunoblasts, and plasma cells. Moreover, benign thymic epithelial cells are present, simulating the B2 subtype of thymoma. The neoplastic cells are positive for CD19, CD20, CD45, PAX-5, and bcl-2 and occasionally for CD43, and they express monoclonal light-chain immunoglobulin. *Primary mediastinal large B-cell lymphoma* is composed of a monomorphic population of large lymphoid cells with abundant cytoplasm and with large irregular, sometimes hyper-lobulated nuclei having small nucleoli. Small clusters of neoplastic cells surrounded by small collagen fibers are usually found. Immunocytochemistry is positive for CD19,

CD20, CD22, CD79a, CD200, PAX-5, Oct2, Bob.1, MAL, and TRAF. Neoplastic cells variably express CD10, CD30, BCL-6, PC-1, and MUM-1. *Anaplastic large-cell lymphoma* usually exhibits large or giant cells, with abundant clear or basophilic cytoplasm and with horseshoe-shaped, kidney-shaped, or cigar-shaped nuclei that have prominent nucleoli (Fig. 5.45). Neoplastic cells usually express CD2, CD4, CD5, CD30 (with membrane and Golgi pattern), CD45, and EMA. Most cases are ALK-positive (Fig. 5.46) and present a t(2;5) or t(1;2) translocation. *Lymphoblastic lymphoma* is composed of small to intermediate-sized lymphoid cells with scant cytoplasm, round or occasionally cleft or convoluted nuclei with a fine and delicate chromatin, and one to three prominent nucleoli. Usually, karyorrhexis, crushing artifact, and cell molding are observed. The B-cell subtype is positive for TdT, CD10, CD19, and PAX-5, and there is cytoplasmic expression of CD20, CD22, CD24, and CD79a. The neoplas-tic cells of the T-cell subtype usually show cytoplasmic CD3, CD7, and TdT and variable expression of CD1a, CD2, CD4, CD5, CD8, CD10, CD34, and CD38. T-cell-receptor gene rearrangements are usually present.

Hodgkin lymphoma   This can originate in the thymus and mediastinal lymph nodes, or it can be secondary, with involve-ment of these organs as part of a diffuse disease; all of the variants of Hodgkin lymphoma can be observed in the medi-astinal lymph nodes. The most common thymic subtype of Hodgkin lymphoma is the nodular sclerosis one; therefore, FNA specimens show scant cellularity, with plasma cells, eosinophils, histiocytes, and the pathognomonic Reed–Sternberg cells and/or the lacunar mononuclear cells arranged in a pseudo-granulomatous pattern. The neoplastic pleomor-phic cells are positive for CD15, CD30, and PAX-5.

5.2.6   Metastases to the Mediastinal Lymph Nodes

Thymus and mediastinal lymph nodes can be secondarily involved by a malignant process either by contiguity (lung, pleura, esophagus, trachea, thoracic wall) or colonization through the hematolymphoid pathway from an intrathoracic or extrathoracic tumor in the lung, larynx, thyroid, breast, kidney, prostate, testis, or ovary. A clinical history of malig-nancy together with imaging studies is important for sup-porting the clinical impression. The cytomorphologic diagnosis can be confirmed by specific immunostainings correlated with those of the primary neoplasm. If the meta-static deposit derives from an unknown primary site, immu-nohistochemistry can be used as described in the previous chapter.

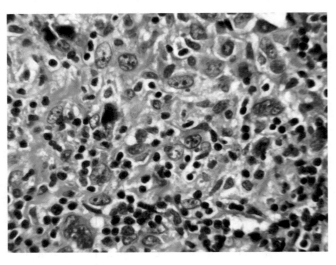

Fig. 5.45 Anaplastic large-cell T-cell lymphoma. H&E (high magnification)

5.3   Chest Wall Masses

There is a wide variety of malignant tumors that involve the chest wall. Primary neoplasms originate from mesothelium, soft tissue, bone, osseocartilaginous tissue, dermis, or subcu-taneous tissue. More than half of secondary chest wall tumors are metastases from distant organs; the rest are the result of direct invasion from adjacent structures, such as the breast, lung, pleura, and mediastinum.

Thoracic wall neoplasms can be classified on the basis of their prevailing cytomorphologic pattern: pleomorphic, spin-dle, epithelioid, biphasic, myxoid, and small round/ovoid. Although some cytomorphologic aspects may suggest the histotype of the lesion or a specific line of differentiation, the definitive diagnosis is carried out by simultaneous evaluation of both the cellular characteristics and the immunocyto-chemical results after the use of an adequate antibody panel.

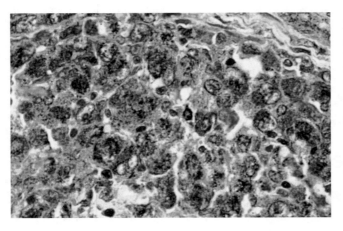

Fig. 5.46 Anaplastic large-cell T-cell lymphoma. ALK immunostain (high magnification)

5.3.1 Pleomorphic Pattern

The cytology of FNA samples usually shows single or grouped cells of variable sizes and shapes.

Pleomorphic leiomyosarcoma Neoplastic cells usually exhibit abundant cytoplasm, nuclear pleomorphism, aniso-karyosis, and multinucleation. Nuclei are hyperchromatic with coarse chromatin. The immunophenotypic profile of this neoplasm is characterized by positivity for vimentin, desmin, α-SMA, smooth muscle myosin, muscle-specific actin (HHF-35), and h-caldesmon. Isolated neoplastic cells immunostained with CD34, S-100 protein, CK8, and CK18 can be observed.

Pleomorphic liposarcoma Cytology smears show moderate to high cellularity with markedly anaplastic and pleomorphic cells and small tumor cell clusters. Large adipocytes of variable nuclear size and shape, ranging from small and compressed to large and round/oval and hyperchromatic, admixed with lipoblasts that have abundant homogeneous to multivacuolated cytoplasm, can be observed. Lipid droplets and bizarre, occasionally scalloped bare nuclei with coarse chromatin and prominent nucleoli can be identified in the background. Neoplastic cells are positive for vimentin and S-100 protein, whereas only occasional spindle elements express CD34. Amplification of the *MDM2* and *CDK4* genes results in expression of MDM2 and CDK4 in some round and pleomorphic cells, and they are immunostained with MDM-2 and CDK-4. Cytogenetics shows increased chromosome numbers with complex rearrangements. Usually there are deletions of chromosome arms 13q and 16q.

Undifferentiated pleomorphic sarcoma Cytology shows high cellularity with variable proportions of cell clusters and with single cells dispersed in a necrotic background. Markedly pleomorphic, spindle-shaped, and/or epithelioid cells with abundant cytoplasm and giant cells with single or multiple nuclei are observed (Fig. 5.47). There are mitoses, sometimes numerous, with atypical forms. Neither cytomorphology nor immunocytochemistry allows identifying or suggesting a differentiation cell line. Neoplastic cells usually express vimentin (Fig. 5.48) and occasionally, in rare cells, cytokeratins, desmin, or EMA. A complex karyotype with marked intratumoral heterogeneity is observed by cytogenetic analysis.

Pleomorphic rhabdomyosarcoma FNA samples show hypercellularity, with usually numerous large, very pleomorphic dispersed cells and occasional small clusters of polygonal cells. A rhabdoid cytomorphology, consisting of cells with abundant cytoplasm and perinuclear globoid density, eccentrically located nuclei, sometimes binucleated and

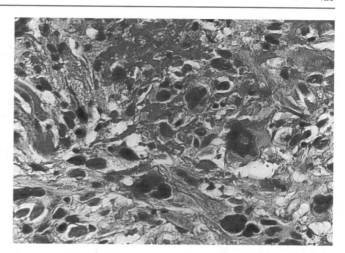

Fig. 5.47 Undifferentiated pleomorphic sarcoma. H&E (high magnification)

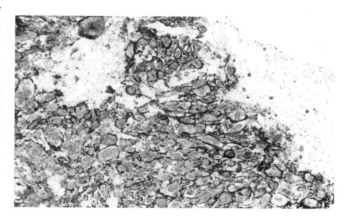

Fig. 5.48 Undifferentiated pleomorphic sarcoma. Vimentin immunostain (high magnification)

multinucleated, with prominent nucleoli, is common. Most undifferentiated cells express only vimentin, whereas, with the progression of differentiation, neoplastic cells begin to express desmin, muscle-specific actin, myogenin, MyoD1, Myf-3, Myf-4, and Myf-5. The most differentiated tumor cells can also be immunostained with antibodies for myoglobin, tropomyosin, striated-muscle myosin, isoenzyme B and M of creatine kinase, titin, acetyl choline receptors, and dystrophin. Occasionally, neoplastic cells can express S-100 protein, CD57, NSE, and CK8.

Pleomorphic carcinoma This poorly differentiated or undifferentiated carcinoma exhibits a mixed population of pleomorphic spindle, large, and/or giant cells without signs of squamous, glandular, mesenchymal, or neuroendocrine differentiation. In cytologic preparations, there are scattered, isolated, strikingly large cells, which are often multinucleated with round nuclei and prominent nucleoli. Immunocytochemistry yields positive results for cytokeratins and vimentin.

Anaplastic large-cell lymphoma FNA cytology is characterized by the presence of pleomorphic intermediate, large, and/or giant cells, and Reed–Sternberg-like cells, with irregular nuclei and one or more nucleoli, in a background of histiocytes and neutrophils. Neoplastic cells are positive for CD2, CD4, CD5, CD30 (with the typical cytoplasmic dot-like immunostaining), CD45, and EMA. Most cases also are positive for ALK and have a t(2;5) or t(1;2) translocation.

5.3.2 Spindle Cell Pattern

This group is composed of tumors characterized by a predominance of spindle cells with elongated cytoplasm and ovoid or fusiform nuclei, usually arranged in sheets or fascicles. Few single cells and some round, polygonal cells with abundant cytoplasm, and nuclei of variable size and shape, may be present.

Leiomyosarcoma Cytology smears usually show tissue fragments with a variable arrangement: closely packed tissue fragments with rigid edges, loosely cohesive clusters, and short fascicles with elongated cells. Neoplastic cells have elongated cytoplasm and centrally located oval or elongated nuclei, with blunt or rounded ends ("cigar-shaped"). Single isolated cells and naked nuclei are often present. Tumor cells have the same immunophenotype as do the pleomorphic variants, i.e., positivity for vimentin, desmin, α-SMA, smooth muscle myosin, muscle-specific actin (HHF-35), and h-caldesmon.

Schwannoma (neurilemmoma) Cytologic preparations are moderately cellular, with cells in cohesive clusters and small fascicles; singly scattered spindle-shaped tumor cells are also present. The neoplastic cells are arranged in syncytium-like fragments and show moderate amounts of filamentous cytoplasm, minimally atypical nuclei that range in shape from oval to wavy to fish-hook-like, and inconspicuous nucleoli. Immunostainings are positive for vimentin, S-100 protein (mainly β-subunit), laminin, and type IV collagen. Some cells express calretinin, calcineurin, CD56, CD57, bcl-2, and NGF-R.

Malignant peripheral nerve sheath tumor (MPNST) FNA cytologic samples are moderately to highly cellular, composed of variably sized cell fascicles, isolated spindle cells, and naked nuclei (Fig. 5.49). The neoplastic cells are relatively large and predominantly oval but may be pleomorphic and/or round. Cancer cells have a scarce, tapered, and fibrillary cytoplasm and undulating or comma-shaped nuclei, sometimes with mild to marked pleomorphism, occasionally being giant, bizarre, and hyperchromatic with prominent or inconspicuous nucleoli. Mitoses, apoptosis, necrosis, and

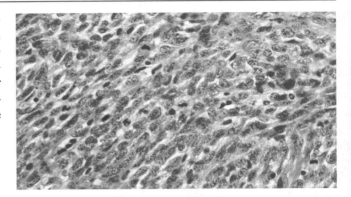

Fig. 5.49 Malignant peripheral nerve sheath tumor. H&E (high magnification)

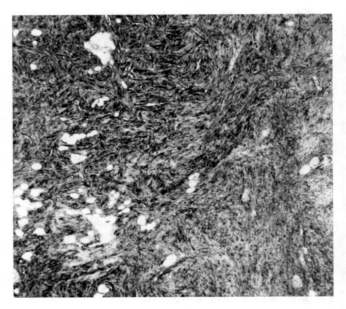

Fig. 5.50 Malignant peripheral nerve sheath tumor. Nestin immunostain (high magnification)

sporadic rosette-like or pseudoglandular cell arrangements may be observed. Immunocytochemistry shows variable cell positivity for S-100 protein, PGP9.5, nestin (Fig. 5.50), SOX2, and HMGA2.

Monophasic synovial sarcoma This variant shows moderate to marked cellularity: single cells are admixed with branching tissue fragments in prominent fascicular and whorled growth patterns (Fig. 5.51). The neoplastic cells have scant and delicate cytoplasm, ovoid to spindled nuclei with evenly distributed bland chromatin, and inconspicuous nucleoli. These cells are positive for vimentin, calponin, bcl-2, CD34, and TLE1 (Fig. 5.52). Some cells may express CD99, calretinin, CD56, CD57, and SYT, with occasional presence of cytokeratins and EMA. Molecular tests show the presence of the chromosomal translocation t(X;18)

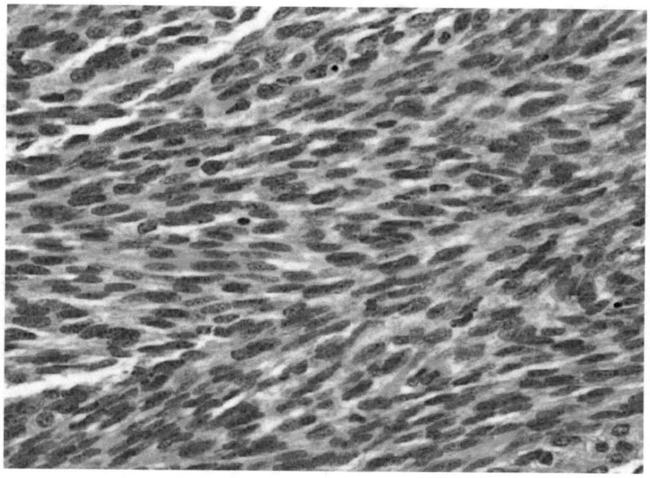

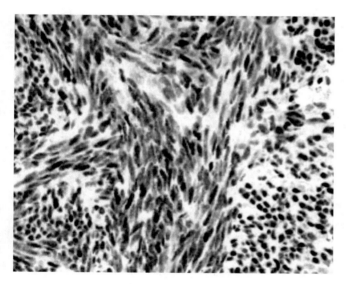

Fig. 5.51 Monophasic synovial sarcoma. H&E (high magnification)

Fig. 5.52 Monophasic synovial sarcoma TLE1 immunostain (high magnification)

(p11;q11), which involves the genes *SSX1*, *SSX2*, or *SSX4* in the X chromosome and the *SYT* gene located on chromosome 18.

Fibrosarcoma This is a rare tumor that, in cytologic FNA samples, shows a proliferation of usually well-differentiated fibroblastic elements that are structured in bundles, fascicular structures, and storiform aggregates. The neoplastic cells are elongated and have little recognizable cytoplasm, fusiform or oval nuclei with slightly coarse chromatin, and inconspicuous or prominent nucleoli. From an immunocytochemistry point of view, immunoreactivity for vimentin, fibronectin, type I collagen, and laminin is observed. Positivity for CD34 is seen only in cases arising in a previous dermatofibroma or in a previous solitary fibrous tumor.

Solitary fibrous tumor FNA cytology shows little or moderate cellularity, with a bloody background that contains tissue fragments with a meshwork of irregular fascicles, isolated spindle-shaped cells, and naked nuclei. The neoplastic cells usually are bland, with scant elongated cytoplasm, fusiform nuclei, finely dispersed chromatin, and inconspicuous nucleoli. The presence of nuclear pleomorphism, prominent nucleoli, necrosis, and noticeable mitotic activity should raise the suspicion of the rare malignant variant. Neoplastic cells have a positive immunophenotype for vimentin, CD34, CD99, factor XIIIa, and bcl-2. The CD10 molecule is also expressed in more than half of the cases, whereas immunostaining for S-100 protein and SMA protein occurs only in a few cells. STAT6 immunostaining is a good surrogate marker that highlights the genetic alteration (*NAB2–STAT6* gene fusion) that is present in the solitary fibrous tumor.

Inflammatory myofibroblastic tumor Cytologic preparations are usually highly cellular and are composed of a mixture of spindle-shaped cells present in isolated form, in loose clusters, and in dense aggregates admixed with an inflammatory cell population of lymphocytes, lymphoplasmacytes, and plasma cells. The spindle cells (myofibroblasts) have cytoplasmic vacuolization as well as cytoplasmic tails, slightly eccentrically placed, plump nuclei with finely granular chromatin, and conspicuous small nucleoli. The neoplastic cells are positive for vimentin, desmin, and/or α-SMA. Immunocytochemistry on the inflammatory lymphoid cell population always reveals a reactive immunophenotypic profile without clonal restrictions. On molecular tests, translocations involving the *ALK* gene on chromosome 2(p23), mainly t(1;2) (q25;p23), t(2;19) (p23;q13), and t(2;17) (p23;q23), are found in this lesion. Because the ALK immunoreactions do not include all the chimeric molecules generated by the various translocations, it is possible to obtain negative results when routine antibodies are used.

Sarcomatoid mesothelioma FNA usually does not yield diagnostic material, and smears are essentially bloody. Occasionally, it is possible to highlight rare, fusiform cells that are isolated or gathered in minute aggregates. Immunocytochemical investigations also are not contributory to the diagnosis, because the classic markers of mesothelioma are expressed only occasionally in the neoplastic cells.

5.3.3   Epithelioid Pattern

This group includes tumors of epithelium-like appearance that, on FNA cytology, shows cohesive neoplastic cell aggregates as well as numerous individually dispersed neoplastic medium-sized or large, round, or polygonal cells with ample cytoplasm and nuclei of variable size and shape.

Epithelioid sarcoma, distal subtype Cytologically, isolated cells admixed with small vaguely cohesive groups of neoplastic cells are observed. The tumor cells are round, polygonal, or spindle-shaped, with moderate to abundant dense, sometimes vacuolated cytoplasm and mildly pleomorphic, large, round, and eccentrically placed nuclei with vesicular, occasionally clumped chromatin and one or more small nucleoli (Fig. 5.53). The neoplastic cells are immunoreactive with vimentin, CK (Fig. 5.54), EMA (Fig. 5.55), and CD34.

Clear-cell sarcoma of soft tissue FNA cytologic preparations show moderate to high cellularity, with mostly isolated cells and occasional small-cell clusters. Neoplastic cells are round, polygonal and fusiform, and of variable size. They

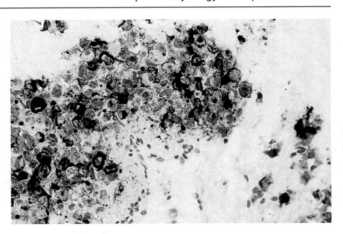

Fig. 5.55 Distal type epithelioid sarcoma. EMA immunostain (high magnification)

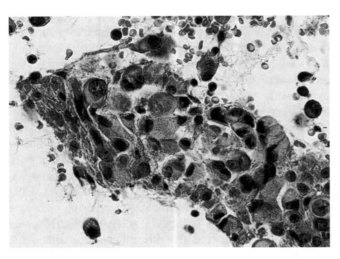

Fig. 5.53 Distal type epithelioid sarcoma. H&E (high magnification)

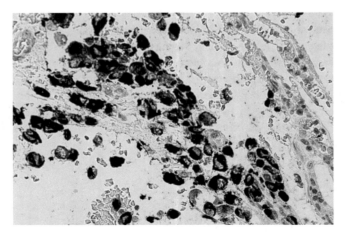

Fig. 5.54 Distal type epithelioid sarcoma. CK immunostain (high magnification)

exhibit a clear and pale, moderately abundant cytoplasm; occasionally finely vacuolated and large, round to oval, and eccentrically placed uniform, slightly hyperchromatic nuclei with finely granular, irregularly distributed, vesicular chromatin; and usually one central and prominent nucleolus. Intranuclear cytoplasmic pseudoinclusions and binucleated cells are occasionally present. Macrophages containing melanin granules may be seen in the background. Immunocytochemical staining is positive for S-100 protein, melan A, and HMB-45. Molecular tests demonstrate the presence of the translocation t(12;22) (q13;q12) with the *AFT1-EWS* gene fusion product.

Alveolar soft part sarcoma FNA smears are moderately cellular and show a background with numerous naked nuclei. Neoplastic cells usually are uniformly round to polygonal with abundant and finely granular, fragile cytoplasm; nuclei are mildly pleomorphic, hyperchromatic, large, round to oval, with vesicular and finely stippled chromatin; the nucleolus is round, prominent, and central. The neoplastic cells are positive for desmin, S-100 protein, and TFE3, which is a chimeric molecule originating from the fusion protein (ASPL-TFE3) produced by the translocation t(11;17) (p13;q25).

Epithelioid angiosarcoma FNA cytologic specimens show a variable cellularity that is secondary to the bloody dilution. The neoplastic cells are mostly non-cohesive and are rarely aggregated in small clusters. Cells are large and round with a finely granular cytoplasm, markedly pleomorphic, and have eccentrically placed nuclei. This neoplasm is immunostained with CD31, CD34, ERG, and FLI1; F8RAg and cytokeratin may react with some cells.

Undifferentiated pleomorphic sarcoma Cytologic preparations may show epithelioid-type elements. The neoplastic cells are large, sometimes giant, with abundant cytoplasm and single or multiple nuclei. The epithelioid cells are positive for vimentin; some cells can react with cytokeratins, desmin, CD68, or EMA.

Epithelioid mesothelioma FNA samples show single cells and sheets of small, medium-sized, and large polygonal cells with well-defined cell borders, a moderate amount of dense cytoplasm, and a central round nucleus with finely granular chromatin. Cells are immunoreactive with vimentin, CK5, CK6, CK7, CK8, CK18, CK19, calretinin, WT-1, EMA, HMFGP, HBME-1, mesothelin, GLUT-1, and podoplanin. Some cells express CK4, CK14, CK17, AMAD-2, CD44H, N-cadherin, and thrombomodulin.

Anaplastic large-cell lymphoma This lymphoma can involve the chest wall in cases of its systemic spreading. Sometimes, the lesion is characterized by a prevalent epithelioid pattern composed of large cells with a Reed–Sternberg-cell-like appearance. These cells show positivity for CD2, CD4, CD5, CD30, CD45, and EMA. The typical t(2;5) or t(1;2) translocation can be highlighted by use of ALK antibodies.

Melanoma This malignancy also can involve the chest wall and can assume a prevalent epithelioid appearance. Neoplastic cells are dispersed or arranged in loose clusters and usually lack melanin pigment in their cytoplasm, which sometimes appears vacuolated, abundant, and poorly defined; nuclei are eccentrically placed, large, and of variable size and shape; binucleation, intranuclear pseudoinclusions, and two or more conspicuous nucleoli or a single prominent nucleolus are observed. Immunocytochemistry shows positivity for S-100 protein, melan A, HMB-45, and SOX-10.

Carcinoma Breast and lung carcinomas can infiltrate the chest wall by contiguity or as metastatic deposits. Breast carcinoma shows a cytomorphology that is similar to that of the primary tumor. Immunocytochemically, it is characterized by positivity to GATA-3, CK7, CK8, CK18, CK19, and a variable presence of mammaglobin, GCDFP-15, ER, PgR, and HER-2. E-cadherin is expressed in the ductal subtype and p120 protein in the lobular subtype. Metastases from lung cancer are derived mainly from adenocarcinoma, which usually shows a poorly differentiated cytomorphology; metastatic cells are positive for CK7, TTF-1, and/or napsin A, EMA, CEA, ERA, ESA, and B72.3.

5.3.4 Myxoid Pattern

The various myxoid soft tissue lesions are characterized by a subfloor consisting of an amorphous, abundant, and homo-geneous myxoid matrix, which takes on a different color depending on the type of staining performed. The diagnosis of myxoid lesions can be suggested based on the cytomorphologic aspects, but the definitive diagnosis should be made subsequent to the results of immunostains and/or molecular biology investigations.

Fibromyxoid sarcoma The FNA cytologic preparations show rare, slightly pleomorphic, isolated spindle cells, naked nuclei, and collagen fibers, which are admixed with small clusters of round/polygonal/spindle-shaped cells, all embedded in a collagenous and myxoid matrix. The cytomorphology does not allow a confident diagnosis of this neoplasm or its differentiation from similar myxoid lesions. However, high-grade sarcoma can be excluded. Immunocytochemistry can be helpful, because MUC4 immunostaining is a marker of this neoplasm. Another diagnostic aid for obtaining a correct diagnosis is the presence of a t(7;16) (q34;p11) translocation.

Myxoid liposarcoma Cytologic samples are moderately to markedly cellular, with a strikingly monotonous appearance. In the low-grade subtype, numerous round to oval tumor cells with scant cytoplasm and indistinct cell borders admixed with tissue fragments of myxoid stroma and thin-walled vessels are observed. The lipoblasts are usually small and uni- or bivacuolated, resembling signet-ring cells. In high-grade tumors, there are numerous isolated and clustered, rarely vacuolated cells with scant cytoplasm, centrally placed nuclei with vesicular chromatin, and multiple, prominent nucleoli. Immunocytochemistry is positive for vimentin, S-100 protein, and TLS in both subtypes. A molecular biology assessment for the presence of a t(12;16) (q13;p11) or t(12;22) (q13;q12) translocation helps one to distinguish this neoplasm from other myxoid lesions.

5.3.5 Small Round/Ovoid Cell Pattern

Most neoplasms included in this group are tumors affecting children and young adult patients and are high-grade malignancies.

Extraskeletal Ewing sarcoma FNA cytologic preparations are highly cellular and show predominantly isolated cells, scattered small cohesive clusters, and numerous naked nuclei. The neoplastic cells are of small to medium size with ill-defined cytoplasmic borders, scant cytoplasm with small intracytoplasmic vacuoles, and round to oval nuclei with prominent nuclear molding (Fig. 5.56). Tumor cells express CD99 (Fig. 5.57) and FLI-1 (Fig. 5.58). Molecular or cytogenetic investigations for documenting the translocation t(11; 22) (q24; q12) or similar gene alterations leading to

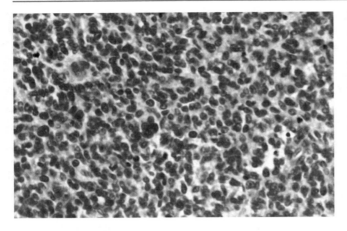

Fig. 5.56 Ewing sarcoma. H&E (high magnification)

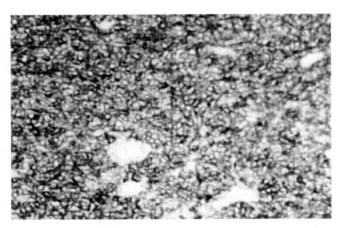

Fig. 5.57 Ewing sarcoma. CD99 immunostain (high magnification)

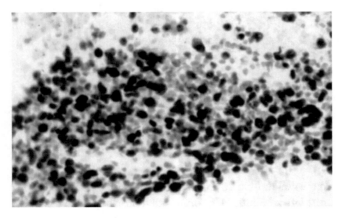

Fig. 5.58 Ewing sarcoma. FLI-1 immunostain (high magnification)

fusion products with the *FLI-1* gene are necessary for confirmation of the diagnosis.

Desmoplastic small round cell tumor Cytology samples show variable cellularity, with sheets and clusters of loosely cohesive small to intermediate-sized cells, uniformly undifferentiated, and predominantly round to oval, with rare polygonal or spindled forms. Cells have a scant, pale, and amphophilic to eosinophilic cytoplasm. Nuclear molding may be present. Nuclei are hyperchromatic, with finely granular chromatin; nucleoli are inconspicuous. Occasional isolated cells are present among fragments of collagenous (desmoplastic) stroma. The tumor cells are immunoreactive for CK-LMW (except for CK7), vimentin, and WT-1. Desmin is usually positive, with a dot-like cytoplasmic pattern. Some cells may express EMA, NSE, and CD99. Molecular analysis, including FISH, identifies the characteristic translocation t(11; 22) (p13; q12), which results from the fusion of the *EWS* gene (Ewing sarcoma gene) located in 22q12 and of the gene *WT-1* (Wilms tumor gene) mapped at 11p13.

Rhabdomyosarcoma The FNA cytomorphology and immunocytochemical profile do not allow one to distinguish between the embryonal and alveolar variants. Therefore, the use of molecular investigations is necessary, because the two variants have different prognostic aspects. *Embryonal rhabdomyosarcoma* FNA samples are moderately to highly cellular and are composed predominantly of isolated cells and occasional loose aggregates. Cancer cells vary from small to intermediate-sized; they are round, polygonal, or spindleshaped. The larger cells show rhabdomyoblast differentiation, with a belt- or tadpole-shaped, elongated cytoplasm and eccentric nuclei with dense hyperchromatic chromatin and irregular nuclear membranes. *Alveolar rhabdomyosarcoma* shows a larger number of round neoplastic cells, with larger and more irregular nuclei, variable presence of rhabdomyoblasts, and multinucleated giant cells, as compared to the embryonal variant. The two variants show the same immunophenotypic profile: the less differentiated neoplastic cells are positive for vimentin, desmin, muscle-specific actin, myogenin, MyoD1, Myf-3, Myf-4, and Myf-5. The most differentiated tumor cells can also be immunostained with antibodies for myoglobin, tropomyosin, striated muscle myosin, and isoenzymes B and M of creatine kinase. Cytogenetic investigations show trisomies 2q, 8, and 20 and loss of heterozygosity at 11p15 in the embryonal variant. Translocation t(2;13) (q35; q14) with production of chimeric PAX3-FOXO1 protein, or translocation t(1;13) (p36; q14) with production of PAX7-FOXO fusion protein, can be detected in the alveolar variant. In this subtype, it is also possible to observe immunostaining for PAX-3 or PAX-7 in some neoplastic cells.

5.4   Intramural Masses of the Gastrointestinal Tract

Sub-epithelial (intramural) masses are usually found randomly during endoscopic or radiologic investigations (barium contrast radiography, magnetic resonance imaging, or computed tomography of the abdomen). These masses are mostly non-epithelial and may originate from any layer of the gastrointestinal (GI) tract wall. Endoscopic ultrasound (EUS) can characterize these masses by identifying the layer of origin; cell and tissue samples can be harvested by means of EUS-guided FNA. A presumptive differential diagnosis of an intramural mass can be made based on the location in the GI tract (esophagus, stomach, small bowel, and colorectum), the GI wall layer of origin assessed by EUS, and on cytomorphology. Besides cytomorphologic evaluation, immunohistochemical, flow cytometry, and molecular diagnostic analysis can be performed on the cytologic samples. The most frequent gastrointestinal intramural neoformations are mesenchymal neoplasms (gastrointestinal stromal tumor, Schwannoma, smooth muscle, and adipose tissue) and lymphomas.

5.4.1   Gastrointestinal Stromal Tumor (GIST)

This tumor is commonly found in the stomach and in the colorectum. The cytologic FNA preparations may show three different patterns: (1) spindle cell (Fig. 5.59); (2) epithelioid; and (3) mixed, consisting of spindle and epithelioid cells. The neoplastic spindle cells are present in tight aggregates with irregular borders and are focally palisading with ill-defined cytoplasmic borders. Variable numbers of loosely cohesive cells are mainly found in epithelioid GIST and at the edges of spindle cell GIST. The nuclei are spindle-shaped or ovoid, with fine and evenly distributed chromatin and

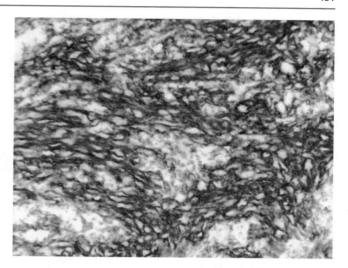

Fig. 5.60   GIST. CD34 immunostain (high magnification)

inconspicuous nucleoli. Spindle cell GIST cannot be distinguished from Schwannoma by cytomorphology only; immunocytochemistry is crucial for making this distinction. GIST is positive for CD117 (c-kit), DOG-1, vimentin, CD34 (Fig. 5.60), and PDGF-R.

5.4.2   Leiomyoma/Leiomyosarcoma

These smooth muscle neoplasms are rare and are found mostly in the esophagus. The cytomorphologic features of FNA samples include the presence of cohesive and well-structured spindle cells showing scant to moderate cytoplasm without clear cytoplasmic borders, "cigar-shaped" nuclei, and fine, evenly distributed chromatin. Hypercellularity, pleomorphism, and mitoses are observed in malignant lesions. Malignant and benign tumors are positive for vimentin, desmin, α-SMA, smooth muscle myosin, muscle-specific actin (HHF-35), and h-caldesmon.

5.4.3   Glomus Tumor

Glomus tumor is a rare soft tissue tumor, generally benign, that involves mainly the stomach, particularly the antrum. FNA cytologic preparations show moderate cellularity, with tightly cohesive cell clusters and single scattered neoplastic cells, vascular endothelial cells, and smooth muscle bundles. The neoplastic cells are small, uniform, and round, with a small amount of cytoplasm and relatively round nuclei. Some elements exhibit a clear cytoplasm. Immunostainings are positive for vimentin, αSMA, h-caldesmon, and calponin. Another characteristic is the staining of cell membranes with laminin and type IV collagen.

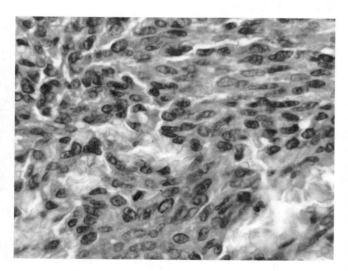

Fig. 5.59   GIST. H&E (high magnification)

5.4.4   Schwannoma

This is a rare, benign tumor predominantly located in the stomach. FNA cytology shows spindle-shaped cells arranged in interlacing fascicles separated by myxoid or hyaline stroma. The neoplastic cells have poorly defined eosinophilic cytoplasm and often wavy, bland-appearing, elongated, thin nuclei. The neoplastic cells are immunoreactive with vimentin, S-100 protein, nestin, calretinin, CD56, laminin, and NSE.

5.4.5   Granular Cell Tumor

Granular cell tumors are rare, benign tumors, which are mainly located in the esophagus, whereas involvement in other gastrointestinal locations such as the stomach or large and small intestine is uncommon. Cytology shows single cells and clusters of cells with ill-defined margins, eosinophilic cytoplasm, and large round to oval nuclei. The neoplasm originates from Schwann cells and therefore exhibits the same immunocytochemical profile as does schwannoma.

5.4.6   Lipoma

Submucosal lipomas are more frequent than are liposarcomas. The FNA cytology of lipoma shows small fragments of mature adipocytes with vacuolated cytoplasm and peripheral oval and uniform nuclei. Immunocytochemical stains (vimentin and S-100 protein) usually are not necessary for making the diagnosis.

5.4.7   Liposarcoma

This tumor is exceptionally rare as a primary neoplasm of the gastrointestinal tract; it is usually a secondary involvement from a tumor originating in the retroperitoneum. FNA cytologic features depend of the subtype of liposarcoma.

Well-differentiated subtype This tumor is composed of small fragments of fatty tissue similar to those of lipoma, but nuclear atypia and lipoblasts are present. Well-differentiated liposarcomas express vimentin, S-100 protein, MDM-2, and CDK-4.

Pleomorphic subtype This tumor shows large adipocytes with abundant homogeneous or multivacuolated cytoplasm, variable nuclear size and shape, and prominent nucleoli; lipoblasts are also present. In contrast to well-differentiated liposarcoma, the pleomorphic and dedifferentiated subtypes express occasional immunoreactivity.

5.4.8   Vascular Tissue Tumors

Hemangioma Gastric and intestinal hemangiomas are very rare lesions. The FNA samples show hemorrhagic aspirates that include rare single cells or small clusters of spindle cells with thin cytoplasmic processes and elongated nuclei, admixed with some siderophages. Immunocytochemistry usually is not necessary; however, if carried out, it shows positivity for vimentin, FVIIIRAg, CD31, CD34, and Fli-1.

Angiosarcoma This rarely occurs in the gastrointestinal tract; however, when present, it usually shows the features of the epithelioid variant. The cytologic preparations are bloody and exhibit large neoplastic cells with cuboidal shape, finely granular abundant cytoplasm, and pleomorphic nuclei. The tumor has the immunophenotype of hemangioma.

Kaposi's sarcoma This is a malignant vascular tumor that occurs in immunosuppressed patients; it is related to human herpes virus 8 (HHV-8) infections. Cytologically, fusiform cells arranged in pseudovascular structures, small clusters, and also singly are observed. Cells show an ill-defined cytoplasmic outline and distorted nuclei. Inflammatory cells and histiocytes are abundant; some of these contain hemosiderin cytoplasmic pigment. Immunocytochemically, the neoplasm shows positivity for vimentin, CD34, CD141 (thrombomodulin), latent nuclear antigen 1 of the herpes virus 8 (HHV-8 LNA-1), and FLI-1. In most cases, CD31 expression is also observed.

5.4.9   Lymphoma

Most gastrointestinal tract non-Hodgkin lymphomas occur in the stomach. Almost any histotype of malignant lymphoma may occur, the vast majority being B-cell lymphomas. The most common varieties are extranodal MALToma, large-cell B-cell lymphoma, and anaplastic lymphoma. Enteropathy-associated T-cell lymphoma may be encountered in the small intestine.

MALT lymphoma FNA cytology shows the same features of MALT lymphomas as those present in other extranodal sites, including a monotonous proliferation of small to medium-sized lymphoid cells with scant cytoplasm and minimal nuclear irregularities. MALT lymphoma cells are positive for CD20, CD19, CD43, CD79a, PAX-5, and monoclonal immunoglobulin light chain. Molecular biology reveals a t(11;18) (q21;q21) translocation.

Large-cell B-cell lymphoma This may present de novo or be due to transformation/progression of a MALT lymphoma. The entire range of molecular variants may be observed, mostly the activated B-cell (ABC) variant. Cytologically, this lymphoma is made up of large atypical lymphoid cells with moderate to abundant cytoplasm, irregular nuclear membranes, vesicular chromatin, and one or multiple prominent nucleoli. Immunocytochemistry is positive for CD19, CD20, CD79a, and PAX-5. The germinal center B-cell (GCB) variant expresses CD10 and/or bcl-6 and lacks MUM1, whereas the ABC subtype is MUM1-positive and CD10-negative, with variable bcl-6 expression. Gene rearrangement of *c-myc*, *bcl-2*, and/or *bcl-6* highlights the "two hit" or the "three hit" variant.

Anaplastic large-cell lymphoma This is composed of large or giant cells with large clear or basophilic cytoplasm and characteristic polymorphous convoluted nuclei with prominent nucleoli. Neoplastic cells usually express CD2, CD4, CD5, CD30, CD45, and EMA. Cases with a t(2;5) or t(1;2) translocation are also ALK-positive.

Enteropathy T-cell-associated lymphoma This rare lymphoproliferative disease occurs in the small intestine, mainly the duodenum. Cytology smears of the neoplastic mass show monomorphic small to medium-sized lymphocytes with moderate to abundant pale cytoplasm, round or angulated vesicular nuclei, and prominent nucleoli (Fig. 5.61). The neoplastic cells show positivity for CD2, CD3, CD7, CD103 (Fig. 5.62), TIA-1, and granzyme B. Some cases also exhibit immunostaining with CD8 and CD56.

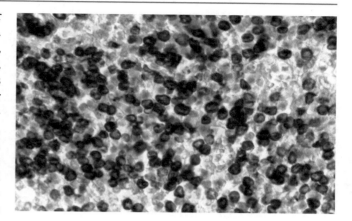

Fig. 5.62 Enteropathy T-cell-associated lymphoma. CD103 immunostain (high magnification)

5.5 Pancreatic Masses

Percutaneous FNA cytology of pancreatic masses is carried out with ultrasound or computed tomography (CT) guidance. Currently, EUS-guided FNA is the most widely used procedure because it offers a great advantage of sampling of small deep-seated lesions compared to other techniques. It also permits a better definition of the location of the mass.

5.5.1 Ductal Adenocarcinoma

Cytologic preparations are usually cellular and are composed of some dispersed cells, cell sheets, and aggregates with variable honeycomb-arranged features. The well-differentiated subtypes have a tendency to retain a flat honeycomb arrangement that is very much akin to the benign pancreatic epithelium. The high-grade subtype shows disorganization of the clusters with loss of cell polarity. Neoplastic cells have moderate amounts of cytoplasm and occasional mucin vacuoles. Nuclei often have irregular chromatin with hypo- and hyperchromasia; the nucleoli are prominent. The nuclear membranes are irregular, with notches, convolutions, and grooves; these are seen mostly in high-grade tumors. Some cells show squamous differentiation. The neoplastic cells express CK7, CK8, CK18, CK19, EMA, DUPAN-2, CEA, CEACAM-1, CD44v6, E cadherin, claudin 18, and annexin A8. A few cells are positive for CK17, CK20, EGF-R, HER-2, and TGF-α. The squamous-differentiated cells can be highlighted with use of antibodies for CK4, CK5, CK13, and p63, whereas the mucin molecules that are occasionally present can react with MUC1, MUC3, MUC4, MUC5AC, CA19.9, CA125, and TAG 72 (B72.3).

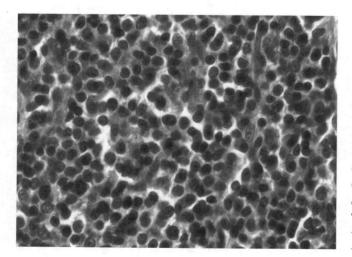

Fig. 5.61 Enteropathy T-cell-associated lymphoma. H&E (high magnification)

5.5.2 Pleomorphic Giant Cell Carcinoma

FNA cytology samples are highly cellular, usually with isolated, pleomorphic, and giant single cells that have round, oval, or spindle shapes. Neoplastic cells have a relatively abundant cytoplasm and single or multiple nuclei. In some cases, phagocytosis of inflammatory cells by tumor giant cells may be observed. Immunocytochemistry is positive for vimentin; some cells express weak positivity with CK7, CK8, CK18, CK19, CEA, and DUPAN-2.

5.5.3 Acinar Cell Carcinoma

FNA cytology shows small cohesive nests of tumor cells in the typical acinar arrangement and many dispersed cells. The tumor cells usually have an eosinophilic and granular cytoplasm, round or oval peripherally placed nuclei, and prominent nucleoli. The neoplasm is immunopositive for CK8, CK18, trypsin, chymotrypsin, α-1-antitrypsin, α-1-antichymotrypsin, lipase, phospholipase A2, and PSTI. Some cells express EMA, CEA, B72.3, MUC5AC, CA19-9, CA125, and DUPAN-2.

5.5.4 Neuroendocrine Tumors

The FNA samples show hypercellularity with discohesive, isolated cells, occasional rosette-like formations, and loose cell clusters. The neoplastic cells are monotonous and small to medium-sized, with plasmacytoid-like morphology and occasional pleomorphism. They have scant to moderate cytoplasm; round to oval, central or eccentrically placed nuclei with the characteristic "salt-and-pepper" chromatin; and no distinct nucleoli. The neoplasm is immunoreactive with the usual neuroendocrine markers, such as chromogranin, synaptophysin, and CD56.

5.5.5 Solid Pseudopapillary Neoplasm

The FNA cytologic preparations appear highly cellular and are composed of numerous non-mucinous cuboidal cells that are both isolated and arranged in loosely cohesive aggregates and single or multiple layers surrounding vascular structures expanded by myxoid or hyaline metachromatic material. Neoplastic cells are cuboidal, with moderate amounts of delicate vacuolated cytoplasm with indistinct cell borders and monomorphic round to oval and sometimes grooved nuclei that have fine granular chromatin, smooth nuclear contours, and indistinct nucleoli. Immunocytochemistry is positive for vimentin, α1-antitrypsin, α1-antichymotrypsin, PgR, CD56, CD10, CD117, and nuclear β-catenin.

Cytokeratins may be positive but usually with weak immunostaining.

5.5.6 Mucin-Producing Cystic Neoplastic Lesions

Mucinous cystic neoplasm FNA samples show variable, usually sparse cellularity, related to the grade of dysplasia, and a background of abundant mucin. Cytologic features are characterized by small clusters and honeycombed sheets of relatively bland mucin-containing columnar cells which can have varying grades of architectural and cytologic atypia. Sheets and groups of benign-appearing mucinous epithelium are observed in low-grade dysplasia; the cells have a vacuolated cytoplasm containing mucin and nuclei with regular nuclear membranes, fine chromatin, and inconspicuous nucleoli. Small, tight, bud-like clustered or isolated cells with a high nucleus/cytoplasm ratio, variably vacuolated cytoplasm, and nuclei with irregular nuclear membranes are observed in high-grade dysplasia. Groups of cells with marked anisonucleosis, as well as nuclei with irregular nuclear membranes and prominent nucleoli, are seen in malignant lesions; cellular debris and necrosis are present in the background. The neoplastic cells express CK7, CK8, CK18, CK19, EMA, CEA, MUC5AC, DUPAN-2, CA19.9, and sometimes MUC-2. In low-grade dysplasia, the marker SMAD4/DPC4 is positive, whereas MUC-1 is negative. In high-grade dysplasia and malignant lesions, SMAD4/DPC4 is absent, whereas MUC-1 is expressed.

Intraductal papillary mucinous neoplasm (IPMN) The WHO considers three groups of IPMN, related to the ducts where the epithelial proliferation occurs: main, branch, and mixed pancreatic ducts. Also, this lesion can have four different histologic types: gastric, intestinal, pancreatobiliary, and oncocytic. The variants except for the oncocytic type show cytomorphologic features similar to those of the mucin-producing cystic neoplastic lesions; therefore, the differentiation between these two entities is based on correlation with clinical and EUS findings. The oncocytic variant is made up of cells with abundant eosinophilic granular cytoplasm and prominent central nucleoli. All subtypes are positive for CK7, CK19, TAG B72.3, and SMAD4/DPC4. Sometimes, the use of some immunocytochemical markers can help one differentiate among the variants. The gastric type is positive for MUC5AC and MUC6; the intestinal type expresses MUC-2, MUC5AC, and CDX-2; the pancreatobiliary type is immunoreactive with MUC-1, MUC5AC, MUC-6, and p53 and in few cells with CEA; the oncocytic type, in addition to expressing mitochondrial antigens, is positive for MUC5AC and MUC-6. HER-2 and EGF-R are also present in IPMN with high-grade dysplasia and carcinoma.

5.6 Liver Masses

Most liver single or multiple mass lesions discovered by palpation or by imaging techniques (nuclear scan, computed tomography, or ultrasonography) are amenable to being sampled by FNA. It is important to establish whether a mass is primary or metastatic; in the latter instance, the harvested sample will be invaluable for cytomorphologic evaluation and immunostaining for help in the search for the primary site, if it is unknown.

5.6.1 Hepatic Adenoma

The FNA cytologic preparations are cellular and show three-dimensional aggregates of hepatocytes with the cytomorphologic appearance of normal cells and numerous stripped, single nuclei. The cells have an abundant granular cytoplasm, sometimes with biliary pigment or fatty changes, and regular round nuclei with smooth borders and a relatively prominent nucleolus. Endothelial cells or fragments of vascular structures may be found along with the hepatocyte aggregates. The lesion expresses the normal hepatocyte markers, such as CK8, CK18, HepPar1, cytoplasmic TTF-1, and ARG-1. CD31 and CD34 can highlight the presence of endothelial elements.

5.6.2 Hepatocellular Carcinoma (HCC)

Well- and moderately differentiated HCC Cytologic samples often show variable numbers of dispersed neoplastic cells, thick trabeculae often outlined by flattened endothelial cells, acinar aggregates, and naked nuclei. The monomorphic neoplastic cells usually have moderate to abundant granular cytoplasm; round, centrally placed nuclei with occasional pseudoinclusions; and prominent nucleoli (Fig. 5.63). Multinucleated cells with nuclear crowding, as well as macronucleoli, may be present.

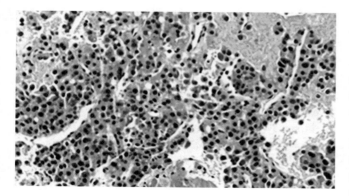

Fig. 5.63 Hepatocellular carcinoma. H&E (high magnification)

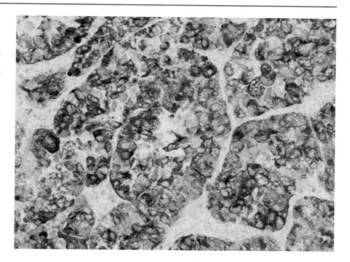

Fig. 5.64 Hepatocellular carcinoma. Glyplican-3 immunostain (high magnification)

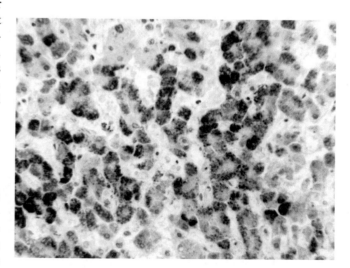

Fig. 5.65 Hepatocellular carcinoma. TTF-1 immunostain (high magnification)

Neoplastic cells are positive for CK8, CK18, HSA, HepPar-1, glypican-3 (Fig. 5.64), and cytoplasmic TTF-1 (only with clone 8G7G3/1) (Fig. 5.65). Some cells may express albumin, α-fetoprotein, ferritin, α-1-antichymotripsin, α-1-antitrypsin, fibrinogen, fibronectin, arginase-1, transferrin receptors, estrogen, and androgen receptors. The endothelial cells may be highlighted with CD31, CD34, and F8RAg. Polyclonal CEA shows only canalicular pattern positivity.

Poorly differentiated HCC Smears show marked cellular anaplasia, including cells with relatively scant cytoplasm, nuclei of various sizes and shapes having coarse chromatin, and irregular single or multiple nucleoli. Atypical naked nuclei may be observed in the background. The immunocytochemical profile is similar to that of well-differentiated HCC; usually HepPar-1 and arginase-1are poorly expressed.

Pleomorphic variant of HCC Cells are large and have abundant cytoplasm, irregular eccentric nuclei, and prominent nucleoli. Multinucleated tumor giant cells are frequently observed. Rare or no trabeculae or bile pigments are seen. The immunocytochemical profile is similar to that of poorly differentiated HCC.

Fibrolamellar variant of HCC This tumor has poor cellularity and exhibits single tumor cells as well as cellular aggregates separated by bundles of fibrous and collagenous fibers together with activated fibroblasts. The neoplastic cells are very large, with abundant oncocytic cytoplasm, sometimes with cytoplasmic invaginations (pale bodies) and hyaline globules. The nuclei are very large and atypical, are centrally located, and show dense granular chromatin with a single giant nucleolus. Immunostainings show positivity for CK7, CK8, CK18, and occasionally CK19, glyplican-3, EMA, CD68, HepPar-1, arginase 1, and albumin.

5.6.3 Cholangiocarcinoma

FNA cytology samples show abundant cellularity composed of cuboidal, columnar, and, sometimes, polygonal neoplastic cells that usually form sheets, three-dimensional clusters, and glandular or acinar structures (Fig. 5.66) and are rarely isolated. Cells have variable amounts of cytoplasm and sometimes vacuolated and polymorphous nuclei with bland chromatin and a conspicuous nucleolus. Nuclear grooves and lobulations can be observed. Immunostaining shows positivity for CK7 (Fig. 5.67), CK8, CK17, CK18, CK19, EMA, CEA, claudin-4, pVHL, MUC5AC, and S100P.

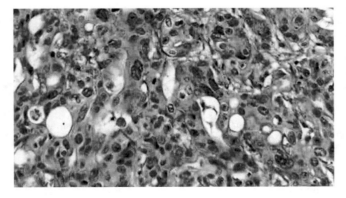

Fig. 5.66 Cholangiocarcinoma. H&E (high magnification)

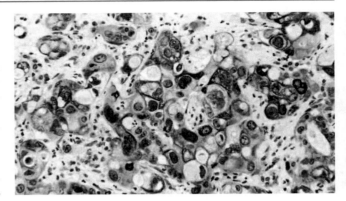

Fig. 5.67 Cholangiocarcinoma. CK7 immunostain (high magnification)

5.6.4 Hepatosplenic Lymphoma

FNA cytology samples from this primary hepatic lymphoproliferative lesion are cellular and show a monomorphic population of medium-sized cells with a moderate amount of eosinophilic cytoplasm and round or slightly indented nuclei, moderately dispersed chromatin, and usually small basophilic nucleoli. The lymphomatous cells are usually immunoreactive for CD2, CD3, CD7, T-cell receptor delta, and cytotoxic markers such as TIA-1 and granzyme B. In most cases, the neoplastic cells express CD8 and sometimes CD16 and CD56.

5.6.5 Metastases to the Liver

Hepatic lesions are often identified during clinical staging of known neoplasms performed by radiologic or ultrasound studies, and FNA represents a rapid and minimally invasive procedure for obtaining the diagnosis. The most frequently metastatic tumor type is carcinoma; it is rarely a sarcoma; the most frequent primary sites include the colorectum, lung, pancreas, stomach, and breast. Melanomas and lymphomas also frequently metastasize to the liver. For sarcomas, the most frequent metastases occur from leiomyosarcoma and GIST. If the metastatic lesion is present in a patient who has an already known neoplasm, the comparison between the histomorphologic features of the primary tumor with the FNA cytologic preparations of the liver lesion often allows for an unequivocal diagnosis and avoids further ancillary investigations. The following summarizes the most helpful confirmatory immunostains for the diagnosis of a liver metastasis when the patient has a known primary site, and the cytology suggests a metastasis from such a primary site.

Colorectal carcinoma Immunocytochemistry for CK7, CK20, and CDX-2.

Lung adenocarcinoma Immunocytochemistry for CK7, TTF-1, and napsin A.

Ductal pancreas carcinoma Immunocytochemistry for CK7, CK17, CK20, and DUPAN-2.

Metastatic gastric carcinoma Immunostainings for CK7 and CK20 have variable expression, but CDX-2, HepPar-1, and pS2 protein positivity allows us to make the correct diagnosis.

Breast carcinoma Metastatic cells, independent of the subtype, are positive for CK7 and GATA-3 and variably positive for mammaglobin and GCFDP-15. Immunocytochemistry for ER, PgR, and HER-2 allows selection of an adequate therapy.

Melanoma Cytologic samples of melanin pigmented cells do not require further immunocytochemical investigations, whereas metastases from non-pigmented forms can be highlighted with the use of immunostaining for S-100 protein, melan-A, HMB-45, and SOX-10.

Leiomyosarcoma The metastatic nodules show positivity for vimentin, desmin, α-SMA, smooth muscle myosin, HHF-35, and h-caldesmon.

Gastrointestinal stromal tumor Metastatic cells are positive for vimentin, CD34, CD117 (c-kit), DOG-1, and PDGF-R.

Lymphoproliferative disease All of the varieties of *lymphoma* and *leukemia* can infiltrate the liver and produce nodular metastatic lesions. Their cytomorphologic features are identical to those present in other sites. Usually, single and dispersed cells are observed. Diffuse large B-cell lymphomas are the most common, whereas small-cell lymphomas (follicular lymphoma, MALT lymphoma, lymphocytic lymphoma/CLL, and mantle cell lymphoma) are less common. About half of peripheral T-cell lymphomas and Hodgkin lymphomas involve the liver. Clinical data on the disease together with immunocytochemistry and flow cytometry investigations are essential for making the correct diagnosis, as referred to in Chap. 4.

Metastasis from unknown primary site If the primary site of a metastatic neoplasm is unknown, the cytologic features may suggest a specific primary site, which, together with the clinical data, allows selection of a limited immunocytochemical panel for determining the final diagnosis (see Tables 4.1, 4.2, 4.3, and 4.4).

5.7 Kidney Masses

FNA of kidney masses is performed for harvesting of samples mainly for cytologic diagnosis and sometimes for performance of ancillary studies, such as immunocytochemistry and cytogenetic or molecular biology. Thus, FNA is a method that allows for an accurate diagnosis and provides guidance for proper patient management.

5.7.1 Benign Kidney Masses

Renal infections Radiologic and ultrasound images of a renal abscess, xanthogranulomatous pyelonephritis, and focal bacterial pyelonephritis can present as a tumor mass simulating malignancy. In such cases, FNA cytology shows numerous neutrophils, isolated and aggregated histiocytes, and multinucleated giant cells. Immunocytochemistry is not necessary; however, in doubtful cases, CD68 immunostaining resolves the diagnostic doubt as to xanthogranulomatous pyelonephritis.

Angiomyolipoma FNA cytology preparations show single and aggregated, elongated smooth muscle-like cells admixed with adipocytes, foamy macrophages, and vascular endothelial cells. The neoplastic cells have ill-defined cytoplasm, round or oval nuclei, and visible nucleoli. Sometimes, bizarre cells may be observed. The immunophenotypic profile is characterized by co-expression of melanocytic markers, such as melan A, HMB-45, tyrosinase, and MITF, and smooth muscle antigens, i.e., α-SMA, specific muscle actin, and calponin. Positivity for ER, PgR, NSE, S-100 protein, CD68, and desmin can be observed.

Oncocytoma Cytology smears show numerous medium-sized, isolated cells with well-demarcated cell borders, abundant eosinophilic granular (mitochondria-rich) cytoplasm, and large, round nuclei with prominent nucleoli (Fig. 5.68). Occasionally, isolated pleomorphic or bizarre nuclei may be present. Immunocytochemistry is positive for CK8, CK18, CK19, E-cadherin, K-cadherin, CD15, CD117 (Fig. 5.69), parvalbumin, mitochondrial markers, and β-defensin-1. Some cells can also express EMA and PAX-2.

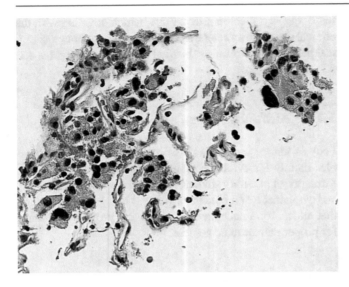

Fig. 5.68 Renal oncocytoma. H&E (high magnification)

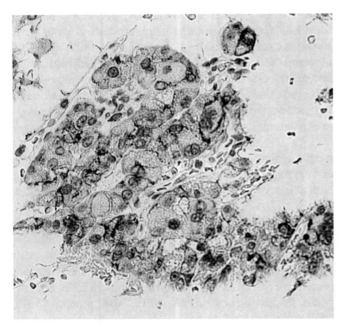

Fig. 5.69 Renal oncocytoma. CD117 immunostain (high magnification)

5.7.2 Malignant Kidney Masses

Clear-cell renal cell carcinoma FNA cytologic specimens show some isolated cells and large tissue fragments. The neoplastic cells have abundant cytoplasm with peripherally placed vacuoles and central granules. Cell membranes are poorly defined. Nuclei are a round to slightly irregular and eccentrically placed, with nucleoli that increase in size in relation to the tumor grade: small and inconspicuous in low grade and prominent in high grade. Immunocytochemistry shows positivity for vimentin, CK8, CK18, CK19, CD10,

RCC, PAX-2, PAX-8, carbonic anhydrase IX, URO-2, URO-3, URO-4, URO-5, URO-10, and villin. Some cells express MUC3, N-cadherin, and aquaporin.

Papillary renal cell carcinoma Cytologically, this tumor is composed of multiple three-dimensional papillary fragments, which exhibit fibrovascular cores covered with cuboid or columnar cells that have scant cytoplasm sometimes containing intracytoplasmic hemosiderin. Nuclei are small and round, frequently grooved, with finely granular and dense chromatin. Nucleoli are small and single, except in high-grade tumors. Neoplastic cells are immunoreactive for CK7, CK8, CK18, CD10, RCC, PAX-1, PAX-8, AMACR, BerEp4, and K-cadherin,

Chromophobe cell renal cell carcinoma FNA samples are usually highly cellular, composed of single cells and usually poorly cohesive cell groups. The neoplastic cells are large and polygonal, and they have abundant clear/pale (in the classic variant) or dense granular eosinophilic (in the eosinophilic variant) cytoplasm. The clear cytoplasm of the classic variant is due to the abundance of microvesicles containing mucopolysaccharides, which provide a vegetable cell appearance and react positively with Hale colloidal iron stain. Nuclei vary significantly in size and occasionally show hyperchromasia, irregular contours and grooves, pseudoinclusions, and binucleation. Immunocytochemistry is positive for CK7, CK8, CK18, PAX-2, PAX-8, CD117, parvalbumin, BerEp4, and E- and K-cadherin.

Collecting duct carcinoma (Bellini tumor) The FNA cytology of this tumor simulates that of a renal metastasis. Smears show single cells and small clusters arranged in papillary configurations. The neoplastic cells have scant dense to vacuolated cytoplasm; large, hyperchromatic nuclei, usually with high-grade atypia; and prominent nucleoli (Fig. 5.70). They are positive for CK7 (Fig. 5.71), CK8, CK18, PAX-8 (Fig. 5.72), and Ber Ep4.

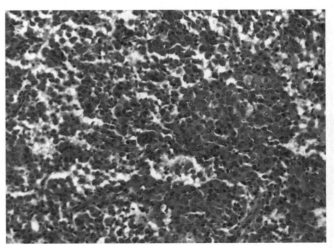

Fig. 5.70 Renal collecting duct carcinoma. H&E (high magnification)

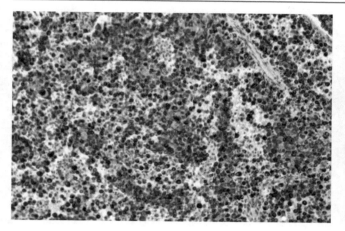

Fig. 5.71 Renal collecting duct carcinoma. CK7 immunostain (high magnification)

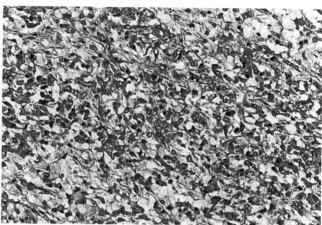

Fig. 5.73 Nephroblastoma. H&E (high magnification)

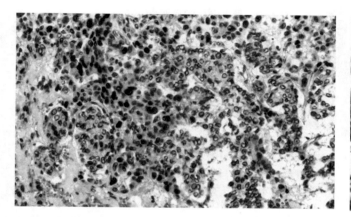

Fig. 5.72 Renal collecting duct carcinoma. PAX-8 immunostain (high magnification)

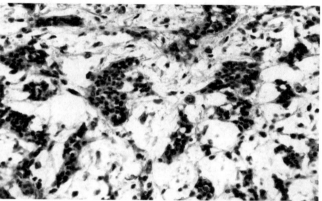

Fig. 5.74 Nephroblastoma. WT-1 immunostain (high magnification)

Xp11.2 translocation-associated renal cell carcinoma This rare tumor shows mixed nested and papillary structures composed of cells with abundant clear and granular cytoplasm, nuclei with vesicular chromatin, and prominent nucleoli. Calcifications are frequent. The neoplastic cells express TFE3, CD10, RCC, PAX-2, PAX-8, and AMACR. Some cells may be positive for CK7, CK8, and CK18.

Mucinous tubular and spindle cell carcinoma FNA preparations of this tumor show a mixture of tubular and aggregated spindle cells of relatively uniform oval to spindle-shaped cells and a background of abundant myxoid matrix. The tumor is positive for CK7, CK8, CK18, PAX-2, PAX-8, AMACR, and EMA.

Nephroblastoma (Wilms tumor) This neoplasm is made up of three distinct cell lines: blastemal, epithelial, and stromal (Fig. 5.73). When at least two of these components are present in the cytologic sample, the cytomorphology suggests the diagnosis; however, when only one cell line is present, the diagnosis can be difficult without the use of ancillary tests. Blastemal cells are small; they have isolated or densely packed with scant cytoplasm, round hyperchromatic overlapping nuclei with finely dispersed granular chromatin, and few prominent nucleoli. Epithelial cells are similar to primitive blastemal elements; they are small with scarce cytoplasm and are often arranged in tubule-like structures, poorly formed tubules, and pseudoglomeruli. Stromal cells are spindle-shaped, sometimes with transversal striations, arranged isolated or in sheets in a loose collagenous stroma. Stromal elements can be smooth or skeletal muscle cells, chondrocytes, adipocytes, or neural. Immunocytochemistry is positive for WT-1 (Fig. 5.74), desmin, and vimentin in blastemal cells. Positivity for WT-1, CK, EMA, and occasionally CD57 is present in epithelial elements. Stromal cells are positive for WT-1 in addition to markers consistent with their origin, i.e., myogenin in rhabdosarcomatous cells and S-100 protein in neural elements.

Urothelial carcinoma Renal–pelvis urothelial carcinomas have the same cytomorphologic features as do the analogous urothelial tumors of the bladder. FNA cytologic preparations of low-grade urothelial carcinoma show isolated single cells, sheets, and/or papillary aggregates composed of columnar or polygonal cells with abundant, moderately dense amphophilic cytoplasm and no vacuolization. Some cells are elongated and may show long cytoplasmic tails with tapered ends. In high-grade tumors, isolated cells and small clusters of large columnar or polygonal cells with scant to moderately dense cytoplasm and large, hyperchromatic irregular nuclei with coarse chromatin are present (Fig. 5.75). Spindle and multinucleated cells and focal squamous differentiation or metaplasia may be seen. The neoplastic cells are positive for CK5, CK7, CK8, CK13, CK17, CK18, CK19, CD141, S100P protein, p63 protein (Fig. 5.76), GATA-3 (Fig. 5.77), and CEA. Some cells can also express CK20, fascin, uroplakin, and nuclear accumulations of p53 protein.

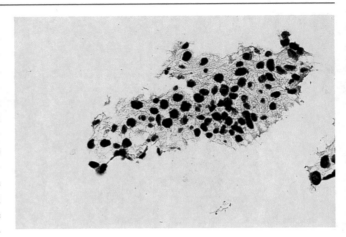

Fig. 5.77 Urothelial carcinoma. GATA-3 immunostain (high magnification)

5.7.3 Metastases to the Kidney

Any histotype of a neoplasm originating elsewhere can potentially metastasize to the kidneys. The most frequent primary sites of renal metastases are the breast, lung, intestine, opposite kidney, and stomach. The kidney may also be involved by contiguity, in particular from carcinomas of the adrenal gland. The knowledge of the clinical data and the morphologic comparison with the primary tumor usually allow one to determine the correct type and origin of the metastatic deposit. However, in doubtful cases, the use of immunostaining contributes to the diagnosis. The characteristics of the secondary neoplasm follow the immunocytochemical profile of the primary neoplasm, as has been described in Chap. 4.

5.8 Adrenal Masses

Currently, all adrenal masses can be cytoaspirated by use of a percutaneous approach under radiologic imaging guidance, i.e., computerized tomography or conventional ultrasound, or, more often, by use of endoscopic ultrasound. FNA is generally avoided when there is a suspicion of pheochromocytoma, as arterial hypertension and more serious complications can occur. Various cytopreparation techniques can be performed with the harvested material; however, the cell block seems the most adequate method for providing material for immunocytochemical investigations.

5.8.1 Benign Adrenal Cortical Nodule/ Adenoma

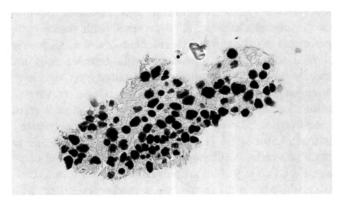

Fig. 5.75 Urothelial carcinoma. H&E (high magnification)

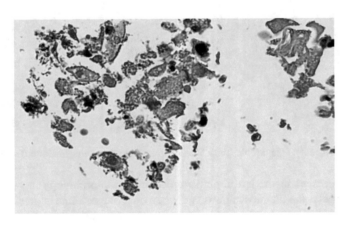

Fig. 5.76 Urothelial carcinoma. p63 immunostain (high magnification)

Here, the cytomorphologic features of the hyperplastic nodules of the adrenal cortex are indistinguishable from those of adrenal adenoma. Therefore, the FNA cytologic diagnosis must include both lesions. Two different cytology patterns may be seen on FNA samples. The first pattern is hypercellular and shows numerous single and aggregated round, small, and naked nuclei seen in a finely vacuolated and granular background due to the fragile cytoplasmic membrane that easily ruptures. The nuclei are uniformly spaced and have an alveolar texture due to their overlap. There are rare cells with intact, lipid-laden cytoplasm. Sparse small spindle cells representing stromal cells can be seen. The second pattern appears less cellular and is composed of discrete aggregates of cells with better-conserved finely vacuolated cytoplasm and round, small, inconspicuous nuclei. Both cytologic patterns show nuclei with fine, uniform, and smooth chromatin, rare intranuclear vacuoles, and inconspicuous nucleoli. Anisonucleosis and features of nuclear pseudo-molding may be present. Nuclear atypia is unusual, and mitosis and necrosis are always absent. The immunophenotypic profile of adenomas and benign hyperplastic cortical nodules is identical. Positive cells for melan A, CD56, inhibin-α, synaptophysin, calretinin, NSE, bcl-2, and vimentin are observed. Occasional cells can express CK8 or CK18. ACTH-positive cells can be observed in adrenocortical hyperplasia with Cushing's syndrome.

5.8.2 Adrenal Myelolipoma

The cytologic samples of FNA are composed of mature adipocytes, immature myeloid cells, erythrocyte precursors, megakaryocytes, and lymphocytes. The immunocytochemistry of the tumor is positive for CD15, CD42a, CD61, CD71, CD68, CD117, CD235a, and myeloperoxidase. The lymphocytes express CD3 or CD20.

5.8.3 Adrenocortical Carcinoma

FNA cytologic preparations show hypercellularity with single and loosely aggregated cells. The well-differentiated variant exhibits a well-defined trabecular pattern or cell sheets with prominent arborizing vessels (Fig. 5.78). Cancer cells have lipid-laden cytoplasm and enlarged hyperchromatic nuclei. Mitosis can occasionally be observed. In the moderately differentiated subtype, the cytoplasm contains fewer lipid vacuoles, is granular, and sometimes shows spherical aggregates resembling rhabdoid bodies. Poorly differentiated carcinoma cells display cellular pleomorphism varying from spindled to polyhedral and sometimes giant, bizarre, and multinucleated forms. The oncocytic variant is composed of polygonal cells with abundant granular and eosinophilic cytoplasm. Independent of the subtype, adrenocortical carcinoma is positive for vimentin and variably posi-

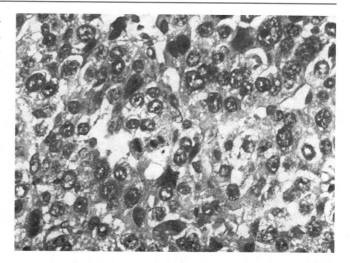

Fig. 5.78 Adrenocortical carcinoma. H&E (high magnification)

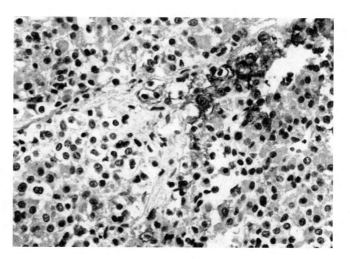

Fig. 5.79 Adrenocortical carcinoma. CK8 immunostain (high magnification)

tive for CK8 (Fig. 5.79) and CK18. Some cells exhibit E-cyclin, IGF-R, l'EGF-R, and sometimes synaptophysin, neurofilament proteins, and NSE.

5.8.4 Pheochromocytoma

FNA cytologic samples are cellular and composed of three different cell types that can be found isolated or combined in loose groups or in pseudo-rosettes. One type of cells is polygonal, small to moderate-sized, with finely granular cytoplasm and uniform round or oval nuclei with granular chromatin (Fig. 5.80). Another cell type is spindle-shaped with abundant cytoplasm and elongated nuclei having coarse granular chromatin. The third type is the myoid-like, with cells which are large, with abundant pale, finely granular

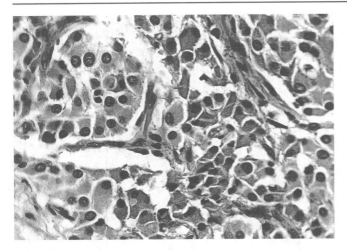

Fig. 5.80 Pheochromocytoma. H&E (high magnification)

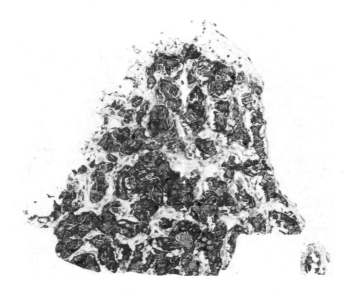

Fig. 5.81 Pheochromocytoma. Synaptophysin immunostain (high magnification)

cytoplasm, eccentric large nuclei, and prominent nucleoli. In cytologic preparations, a mixture of the three cell types can be present, or one type may predominate. Neoplastic cells are positive for immunocytochemical reactions to catecholamines (mainly epinephrine but also serotonin), chromogranin A, synaptophysin (Fig. 5.81), CD56, and NSE. Some cells express bcl-2, GFAP, DOPA, PGP9.5, enkephalin, neuropeptide Y, somatostatin, calcitonin, and ACTH. Only sporadic cells are positive for vimentin, CK8, and CK18.

5.8.5 Neuroblastoma

Cytology preparations show single cells and/or cell clusters forming rosettes with a central fibrillary matrix. Neoplastic cells are small and round, with very scant cytoplasm, dense hyperchromatic nuclei, and coarsely clumped chromatin. Mature or immature ganglion cells may be observed. Neoplastic cells express catecholamine and neuro-associated marker molecules, such as NSE, synaptophysin, calcineurin, and neurofilaments. Some cells are also positive for cathepsin D.

5.8.6 Metastases to the Adrenal Gland

The adrenal glands are a frequent site of metastases, mainly from lung cancer (both small-cell carcinoma and adenocarcinoma). Much less frequently, secondary tumors originate from renal cell carcinoma, gastrointestinal tract carcinomas, lymphoma, and melanoma. The clinical history, correlation with the cytology or histology of the primary tumor, and rational use of immunocytochemical investigations are useful for making the correct diagnosis. Immunostainings of secondary tumors usually maintain the immunophenotypic profile of the primary tumor from which they originate, as was described in Chap. 4.

5.9 Ovarian Masses

The FNA procedure for obtaining cytologic material depends on the size of the lesion, its location, and the available resources (clinical and interventional radiology). FNA material can be harvested by a trans-rectal, trans-vaginal, percutaneous, or during open or laparoscopic surgery. Percutaneous transabdominal FNA can also be performed under imaging guidance. The FNA cytology of the ovary has limitations in not only having a high percentage of false negatives but also and most importantly distinguishing reliably between borderline ovarian tumors and carcinomas. Thus, FNA may be considered unnecessary. In fact, if clinical and imaging investigations suggest a primary malignant ovarian tumor, FNA is often obviated, and surgery is recommended. However, ovarian cytoaspiration can be used for confirming a clinical diagnosis of malignancy in cases of patients who have inoperable ovarian disease or when tumors other than ovarian carcinoma are suspected.

5.9.1 Benign Serous Tumor

FNA cytologic preparations from a benign cystic serous tumor are usually poorly cellular. The occasionally found cyst-lining cells are cuboidal, have uniform round or oval nuclei, and are arranged in crowded groups. Sometimes there are ciliated columnar cells, psammoma bodies, and detached ciliary tufts. The presence of cellular atypia should make one consider the presence of a borderline tumor or carcinoma. If stromal cells are present, it could be an adenofibroma. The neoplasm shows positivity for vimentin, CK7, CK8, CK18, CK19, TAG B72.3, EMA, WT-1, PAX-8, and EpCam. Some neoplastic cells can also be stained with CK4, CK5, ER, and PgR.

5.9.2 Benign Mucinous Tumor

In most cases, the aspirate is cellular and has a gelatinous consistency. The cyst-lining cells are usually isolated or are sometimes arranged in groups or in honeycomb-like sheets. Cells are columnar and resemble benign endocervical or goblet cells. Mucin can be observed in the background and within macrophages. If cellular atypia is present, a borderline tumor or carcinoma should be suspected. The cells show positivity for CK7, CK8, CK18, CK19, TAG B72.3, HAM56, EMA, and EpCam. Some cells are positive for WT-1, mesothelin, CK20, CEA, MUC-2, and MUC-5AC. The intestinal-like cells are immunoreactive for villin, CDX-2, CEA, and CK20 and sometimes for MUC-2 and MUC-5AC. The endocervical-like cells can immunoreact with ER and PgR.

5.9.3 Benign Endometrioid Tumor

FNA cytologic samples show a background of degenerated red blood cells and debris. Occasionally, groups of endometrial-like glandular cells, numerous pigment-laden macrophages, and sometimes some stromal cells are present. Glandular cells are cuboidal to columnar with relatively scant cytoplasm and monomorphic nuclei. Immunocytochemistry is positive for CK7, CK8, CK18, CK19, EMA, and vimentin. Some cells express mesothelin and β-catenin.

5.9.4 Benign Brenner Tumor

Cytologic samples show sheets of urothelial-like cells with oval nuclei and prominent longitudinal nuclear grooves. Sometimes, some fibrous stromal cells are observed. The neoplastic cells are positive for CK7, CK8, CK13, CK18, p63, CEA, URO-3, and CD141. Occasionally, cells are immunoreactive for CK20, whereas the stromal cells are positive for vimentin and bcl-2.

5.9.5 Serous Borderline Tumor and Adenocarcinoma

The FNA cytology of borderline serous tumor and adenocarcinoma is similar. It differs only in the degree of nuclear atypia; therefore, it is not possible to distinguish morphologically between the two lesions. Usually, the cytologic features of the sample include atypical cells in spheres, branching clusters, and sheets. The immunocytochemical profile of these neoplasms is similar to that of the benign tumor.

5.9.6 Mucinous Borderline Tumor and Adenocarcinoma

Cytologic preparations show columnar mucin-producing cells and cells in sheets or arranged in complex aggregates. Nuclei exhibit different levels of atypia; in poorly differentiated cases, they appear intensely pleomorphic. Immunocytochemistry shows the same profile as that seen in benign lesions.

5.9.7 Endometrioid Borderline Tumor and Adenocarcinoma

FNA samples show numerous isolated elongated cells, occasional short cell strips, and intact or fragmented glands with cytomorphologic features of endometrial cells. The background usually is bloody, with hemosiderin-laden macrophages. The neoplastic cells express the antigens of the endometrioid tumors.

5.9.8 Clear-Cell Carcinoma

FNA cytology preparations show a necrotic background in which there are tumor cells with abundant vacuolated or scarce eosinophilic cytoplasm, large pleomorphic and often eccentrically placed nuclei, and prominent nucleoli. Sometimes, hyaline extracellular material is present. The neoplastic cells are positive for CK7, CK8, CK18, CK19, and EMA. Some cells express positivity for CK5, WT-1, OCT-4, CD15, ER, PgR, HNF-1β, and osteopontin.

5.9.9 Mature Teratoma

FNA samples show predominantly anucleated squamous cells, sometimes interspersed with skin adnexal cells, detached ciliary tufts, mucinous cells, and hair fragments. In rare cases, when cystic teratoma has undergone malignant transformation, squamous cell carcinoma is observed. Immunocytochemical investigations are not necessary, because the cytomorphologic pattern is diagnostic per se. Struma ovarii is a particular form of teratoma composed mainly of thyroid elements, including cells with clear or eosinophilic cytoplasm. The immunostains for thyroglobulin and TTF-1 confirm the diagnosis of struma ovarii.

5.9.10 Immature Teratoma

Cytologically, immature teratoma is highly cellular and shows a myxoid background with focal necrosis and hemorrhage. Elements derived from all three layers of germinal tissues are observed cytologically in these tumors. Ectodermal tissue is represented by anucleated, keratinized, intermediate, and parabasal squamous cells. Endodermal tissue is represented by glandular columnar cells which are usually in an acinar pattern. The mesodermal component is characterized by adipose tissue. Particularly represented are neuroectodermal immature elements composed of small round cells with a tendency to form rosettes in a background of neuropil-like material. Immature or embryonic cells are admixed with variable numbers of mature cells. Immunocytochemical reactions follow the cell lineage heterogeneity and correlate with the antigenic distribution of the various tissues represented. Most neoplastic cells usually express vimentin, whereas some cells react with PLAP. Glial cells are positive for GFAP and GFR α-1 (glial-cell-line-derived neurotrophic factor receptor α-1); those of a neurogenic and neuroectodermal nature have immunostaining positive for neurofilaments, NSE, NGF-R, and sometimes synaptophysin. Epithelium-derived cells show positivity for various cytokeratins. Occasional cells express HCG and α-fetoprotein.

5.9.11 Carcinoid Tumors

FNA smears show numerous isolated cells, loose clusters, and occasionally rosettes. Tumor cells have eosinophilic and granular cytoplasm with distinct outlines and an eccentrically placed round or oval nucleus with a granular "salt-and-pepper" chromatin. Intracytoplasmic neurosecretory granules are identified by immunoreactions for chromogranin A and other neuroendocrine markers.

5.9.12 Dysgerminoma

FNA cytology samples are generally hypercellular, and they show a background of small lymphocytes and, in some cases, granulomas, necrosis, and hemorrhage. Neoplastic cells are mainly isolated, with some syncytial loose clusters; clear or granular cytoplasm; large, round, centrally positioned nuclei; and one or more prominent irregularly shaped nucleoli. The neoplastic cells are immunoreactive for PLAP, CD117 (c-kit), SALL4, Oct-3/4 (or Oct-4), D2-40, SOX-17, and NANOG.

5.9.13 Embryonal Carcinoma

FNA cytologic preparations exhibit a monotonous cellular population composed of single cells and sheets of round cells with indistinct, eosinophilic, or pale cytoplasm, round to irregular centrally placed vesicular nuclei, and prominent nucleoli. Cells of bizarre shape and syncytial clusters of anaplastic cells exhibiting pleomorphism and anisonucleosis are seen in some cases. Cancer cells are positive for PLAP, CK, SALL-4, Oct4, NANOG, SOX-2, and CD30.

5.9.14 Yolk Sac Tumor

Cytologic samples are cellular and show isolated neoplastic cells of variable size, loose clusters with occasional glomeruloid structures, and a background of metachromatic mixed mucoid-like material. Cells have a moderate amount of cytoplasm, some cells being vacuolated, and contain intracytoplasmic dense hyaline globules (α-fetoprotein). The nuclei are round to oval with irregular nuclear membranes, coarsely clumped chromatin, and a sometimes inconspicuous nucleolus. Tumor cells express α-fetoprotein, CK, PLAP, SALL-4, SOX-17, and glyplican-3.

5.9.15 Choriocarcinoma

FNA smears usually are hypocellular and show a hemorrhagic background. Scattered large giant cells with a moderate to ample amount of pale or vacuolated cytoplasm and multiple large hyperchromatic and pleomorphic nuclei are present. Most neoplastic cells show expression of vimentin, PLAP, SALL-4, CD10, CK8, CK18, and CK19, whereas only syncytiotrophoblasts show positivity for HCG, inhibin-α, and EGF-R. Some cytotrophoblasts can be immunostained with antibodies to CEA. The intermediate trophoblastic elements are characterized by the presence of CD146 (Mel-CAM) and HLA-G. Some cells express glyplican-3.

5.9.16 Granulosa Cell Tumor

Adult granulosa cell tumor FNA samples are highly cellular, composed of small to medium-sized cells with scant, poorly defined, pale cytoplasm, a monomorphous round or oval and centrally placed nucleus, and pale and finely dispersed chromatin (Fig. 5.82). Naked nuclei and nuclear grooves are usually present.

Juvenile granulosa cell tumor FNA preparations show neoplastic cells that are arranged singly and in loose clusters and exhibit a moderate amount of granular, lipid-rich cytoplasm. The nuclei are round with occasional nuclear protrusions, fine chromatin, and small to prominent nucleoli (Fig. 5.83).

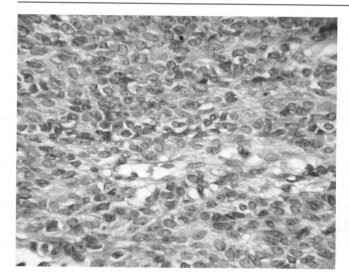

Fig. 5.82 Granulosa cell tumor adult type. H&E (high magnification)

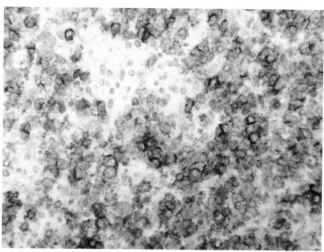

Fig. 5.84 Granulosa cell tumor. CD99 immunostain (high magnification)

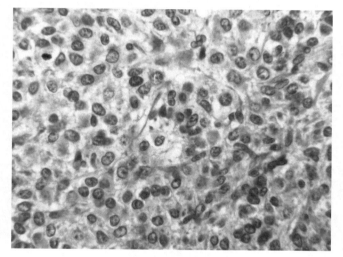

Fig. 5.83 Granulosa cell tumor juvenile type. H&E (high magnification)

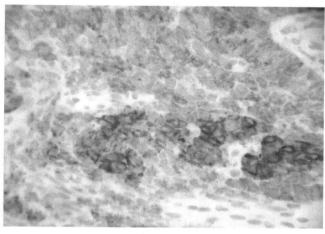

Fig. 5.85 Granulosa cell tumor inhibin-α immunostain. (high magnification)

In both variants, the neoplastic cells are positive for CD99 (Fig. 5.84), inhibin-α (Fig. 5.85), WT1, α-SMA, S-100 protein, ER, PgR, melan A, desmoplakin, SF-1 (steroidogenic factor-1), FOXL2, estradiol, progesterone, and testosterone. CK8 and CK18 may be expressed in a characteristic globular cytoplasmic pattern. Some cells may be immunoreactive with CD56, showing a cytoplasmic immunostaining.

5.9.17 Thecoma

FNA smears are hypocellular and are composed of loose clusters and isolated elongated cells with clear cytoplasm containing lipid vacuoles. The nuclei are spindle-shaped,

with finely granular chromatin. Immunocytochemistry is positive for vimentin, inhibin-α, calretinin, and estradiol.

5.9.18 Fibroma

FNA cytology smears are hypocellular and composed of fibroblastic spindle-shaped bundles of cells similar to those seen in thecoma. Intracytoplasmic lipid is sometimes observed. The cells are positive for vimentin and collagen IV. Some of them express WT-1, SF-1, cytoplasmic CD56, calretinin, muscle actin (HHF-35), and α-SMA.

5.9.19 Metastases to the Ovary

The most common tumors that metastasize the ovaries originate in the gastrointestinal tract (stomach, colon, pancreas, and appendix), breast, female genital tract, and hematopoietic system. Breast lobular carcinomas, including those of the signet-ring cell type, spread to the ovary more frequently than do those of the ductal type. In the absence of clinical data and adequate imaging studies, cytology alone often cannot differentiate between a primary ovarian tumor and a metastasis. The comparison of the cytomorphologic features of a previous neoplasm with those of the ovarian mass can sometimes allow for the correct diagnostic formulation, which can be confirmed with the judicious use of ancillary tests. Even in the case of an unknown primary tumor, immunostaining helps one to determine the diagnosis. In fact, a gastric metastasis shows positivity for CDX-2, HepPar-1, and pS2, with variable immunostaining for CK7 and CK20; colorectum metastatic cells express CK20 and CDX-2; appendix metastases are positive for CK7 and variably for CK20 and CD-2; breast metastases immunoreact with GATA-3 and variably with mammaglobin and GCDFP-15; lymphoproliferative disease cells involving the ovary express lymphoid cell markers and immunoglobulin light-chain restriction or T-cell receptor rearrangement.

5.10 Retroperitoneal Masses

Imaging procedures such as radiography, lymphangiography, fluoroscopy, ultrasound, computed tomography, and magnetic resonance imaging are essential for evaluating retroperitoneal masses and sampling of lesions. Ultrasound offers the greatest advantages, such as relatively low cost, speed of execution, absence of risks from ionizing and magnetic radiation, and no exposure to contrast medium. During harvesting of cytologic material, the tip of the needle can be well visualized, ensuring adequate sampling of the lesion. A range of soft tissue tumors, lymphomas, and metastases can present as retroperitoneal masses in addition to a variety of non-neoplastic conditions.

5.10.1 Retroperitoneal Abscess

Cytologic preparations are characterized by a purulent aspirate composed of a large quantity of intact and partially degenerated neutrophils. Immunocytochemistry is not necessary for diagnosis.

5.10.2 Retroperitoneal Idiopathic Fibrosis

FNA cytologic samples show single spindle cells (fibroblasts) arranged in small fragments, admixed with histio-

cytes, lymphocytes, plasma cells, some eosinophils, and mast cells. A specific diagnosis is possible without immunostainings but with consideration of cytomorphologic features, clinical data, and radiologic findings.

5.10.3 Lipoma and Liposarcoma

The FNA cytology of lipoma shows small fragments of mature adipocytes without nuclear atypia. An atypical lipomatous tumor (well-differentiated liposarcoma) shows cytologic features that are similar to those of lipoma; some adipocytes show nuclear atypia, and a variable number of lipoblasts are present. If there are diagnostic doubts, immunocytochemical reactions for MDM-2 and CDK4 are helpful because they are positive in cases of well-differentiated liposarcoma.

Smears of pleomorphic liposarcoma show large adipocytes with abundant multivacuolated cytoplasm, variable nuclear size and shape, and prominent nucleoli; lipoblasts are also present. Neoplastic cells are positive for vimentin and S-100 protein; only occasional spindle cells express CD34, and some round pleomorphic cells can be immunostained with MDM-2 and CDK4.

Cytologic preparations of dedifferentiated liposarcoma show single cells and clusters of pleomorphic spindle to round cells, occasional multinucleated giant cells, and bizarre-appearing lipoblasts with vacuolated cytoplasm and scalloped nuclei. The liposarcomatous component expresses MDM-2 and CDK4, whereas the heterologous sarcomatous cells mainly express muscle antigens.

5.10.4 Leiomyoma and Leiomyosarcoma

Cytologic specimens of leiomyoma are composed of single and clustered spindle cells with abundant eosinophilic cytoplasm and cigar-shaped nuclei with fine granular chromatin and inconspicuous nucleoli. Leiomyosarcoma usually is a tumor that originates in the uterus and infiltrates the retroperitoneal spaces. It is composed of single and syncytial clusters of spindle cells with abundant cytoplasm and cigar-shaped and blunt-ended atypical nuclei. The two tumors express the same immunocytochemical markers: vimentin, desmin, α-SMA, smooth muscle myosin, muscle-specific actin, and h-caldesmon.

5.10.5 Schwannoma

FNA samples are characterized by numerous single spindle-shaped cells with pale cytoplasm and wavy, elongated nuclei. The neoplastic cells are positive for vimentin, S-100 protein, laminin, and type IV collagen. Some cells can express calretinin, calcineurin, CD56, CD57, bcl-2, and NGF-R.

5.10.6 Malignant Peripheral Nerve Sheath Tumor (MPNST)

Cytology smears show loose cell clusters, fascicular arrangements, and single spindle cells with blunt ends. Neoplastic cells have a scarce and fibrillary, undulating cytoplasm. The nuclei show mild to marked pleomorphism; there are occasional giant, bizarre, and hyperchromatic nuclei and variably present nucleoli. Immunostainings are inconsistent: some cells positive for S-100 protein, PGP9.5, nestin, SOX2, and HMGA2 may be seen.

5.10.7 Undifferentiated Pleomorphic Sarcoma

Smears from this tumor show high cellularity, with single cells and small clusters of markedly pleomorphic, spindle-shaped, and/or epithelioid cells that have abundant cytoplasm and giant cells with single or multiple nuclei. In most cases, immunocytochemistry shows positivity only for vimentin, whereas some cells may occasionally show CK, desmin, and EMA expression.

5.10.8 Proximal-Type Epithelioid Sarcoma

FNA cytologic samples show isolated cells admixed with small, poorly cohesive clusters of round, polygonal, or spindle-shaped cells with a relatively abundant dense cytoplasm, sometimes vacuolated, and large pleomorphic and eccentrically placed nuclei with one or more small nucleoli. The neoplastic cells are immunoreactive with vimentin, CK, EMA, and CD34.

5.10.9 Embryonal Rhabdomyosarcoma

FNA cytology preparations are composed predominantly of isolated cells, with occasional loose aggregates. The neoplastic cells are small to intermediate, round, polygonal, or spindle-shaped. Large rhabdomyoblasts are variably present. The tumor cells are positive for vimentin, desmin, muscle-specific actin, myogenin, MyoD1, Myf-3, Myf-4, and Myf-5.

5.10.10 Extraskeletal Ewing Sarcoma

The tumor shows predominantly isolated cells and scattered cohesive small clusters composed of cells with scant cyto-

plasm, small intracytoplasmic vacuoles, and round to oval nuclei with prominent molding. Numerous naked nuclei are present in the background. Immunoreactions are positive for CD99 and FLI-1. However, cytogenetic studies for documenting the t(11; 22) (q24; q12) or a similar translocation are necessary for confirming the diagnosis.

5.10.11 Malignant Lymphoma

Any type of systemic nodal and extranodal lymphoproliferative disease can infiltrate the retroperitoneal space. Primary retroperitoneal lymphomas are rare and mainly are of high grade, such as diffuse large B-cell lymphoma, Burkitt lymphoma, large-cell anaplastic lymphoma, and lymphoblastic T-cell and B-cell lymphomas. The diagnosis of a lymphoproliferative process is suggested by the cytomorphologic features, but a definitive diagnosis is formulated only with the aid of flow cytometry, immunocytochemistry, and molecular investigations. The cytomorphology of the different types of primary retroperitoneal lymphoma is similar to that of other sites. The cytologic description of these lymphomas and the use of ancillary tests have been described in this chapter and in the previous one.

5.10.12 Metastases to the Retroperitoneum

FNA cytologic samples harvested under image guidance offer a valid diagnostic support in the staging of a known malignancy and avoid unnecessary diagnostic surgery. Metastases of neoplasms of the ovary, uterine cervix, endometrium, vagina, prostate, and gastrointestinal and urinary tracts are frequently diagnosed as being spread to the pelvic and para-aortic lymph nodes. Cytomorphologic features and immunocytochemistry characteristics are similar to their primary counterparts and are reported in different paragraphs of this chapter.

5.11 Central Nervous System (CNS) Masses

Different techniques have been used for obtaining CNS tissue and cytologic material for diagnosis, including open craniotomy, stereotactic-directed FNA, and computed tomography (CT)-guided needle aspiration without stereotactic assistance. Although FNA cytology of visceral organs under radiologic or ultrasound guidance has been widely accepted as a method for rendering a morphologic diagnosis independent of histologic examination, FNA cytology of CNS lesions has not gained uniform acceptance. However, "squash" cytologic preparations can be used for routine intraoperative morphologic diagnosis, and immunocytochemistry on direct smears or on cell blocks can be applied to refine the diagnosis. In addition, harvested material can be submitted to the microbiology laboratory when an infectious lesion is suspected on clinical grounds.

5.11.1 Low-Grade Diffuse Astrocytoma

Cytologically, cellular fragments of fibrillary tissue with a characteristic lumpy appearance are observed. Cells show eosinophilic or faint cytoplasm and sometimes appear as bare nuclei. The nuclei are oval or elongated and have mild atypia, mild to moderate hyperchromasia, and irregular contours (Fig. 5.86). Neoplastic cells are positive for vimentin, GFAP (Fig. 5.87), S-100 protein, and glutamine synthetase. Occasional cells can express CD99, CD56, and HER-2. Immunostaining with antibodies to CD31, CD34, or F8RAg

is of help for better visualization of the possible microvascular proliferation.

5.11.2 Anaplastic Astrocytoma

Compared to low-grade diffuse astrocytoma, the cytologic preparations have greater cellularity, atypia, and mitotic activity. Cancer cells often aggregate to prominent vascular structures. Neoplastic cells have well-defined boundaries and variable cytoplasmic processes, more evident than in low-grade diffuse astrocytoma. The nuclei show atypia, with an increase in size and irregular shape (Fig. 5.88). The immunocytochemistry is analogous to that of low-grade diffuse astrocytoma: positivity for vimentin, GFAP, S-100 protein (Fig. 5.89), and glutamine synthetase.

5.11.3 Diffuse Midline Glioma

This neoplasm is not a variant of astrocytic tumors, but it represents a widely infiltrating glioma expressing a specific

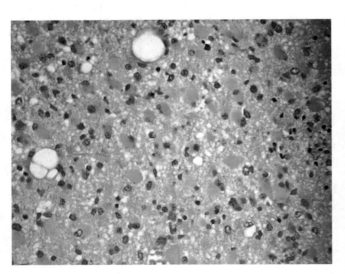

Fig. 5.86 Diffuse astrocytoma. H&E (high magnification)

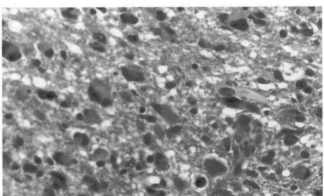

Fig. 5.88 Anaplastic astrocytoma. H&E (high magnification)

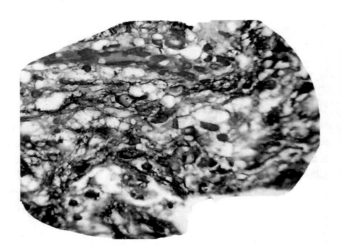

Fig. 5.87 Diffuse astrocytoma. GFAP immunostain (high magnification)

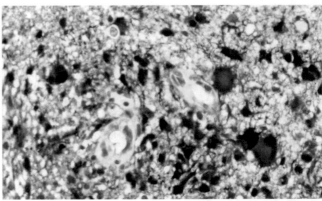

Fig. 5.89 Anaplastic astrocytoma. S-100 protein immunostain (high magnification)

point mutation in the K27 position (codon K27) in the genes coding for histone H3. For identification of this glioma, a specific antibody for the mutant protein K27 M can be used, regardless of whether the protein is derived from mutations in H3F3A or in HIST1H3B/C.

5.11.4 Glioblastoma

Cytologic preparations show a background of necrotic debris that often appears amorphous, sometimes granular, and contains ghost cells and karyorrhectic nuclei. The neoplastic cells are single and discohesive or form small, loose groups that tend to remain close to blood vessels, giving a pseudo-papillary appearance. Tumor cells are anaplastic and have various shapes and sizes: small, large, bizarre, mono- and multinucleated, and with or without nucleolus (Fig. 5.90). The neoplasm is positive for vimentin, GFAP (Fig. 5.91),

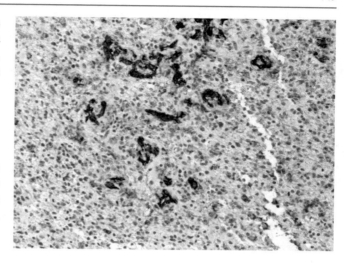

Fig. 5.92 Glioblastoma. CD31 immunostain (high magnification)

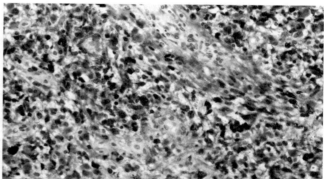

Fig. 5.93 Glioblastoma. IDH1 immunostain (high magnification)

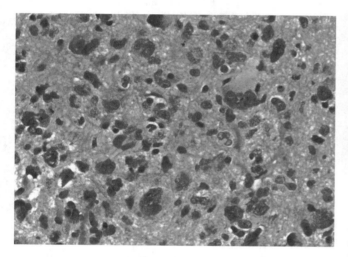

Fig. 5.90 Glioblastoma. H&E (high magnification)

and S-100 protein. Microvascular proliferation can be enhanced by immunostaining for CD31 (Fig. 5.92), CD34, F8RAg, vascular endothelial growth factor (VEGF), collagen IV, and fibronectin. In addition to the conventional immunocytochemistry of glioblastoma, it is important to evaluate other parameters for prognostic and therapeutic purposes. Mutation in the *IDH1* (Fig. 5.93) and/or *IDH2* genes is found only in glioblastoma originating from a low-grade glioma (secondary glioblastoma), whereas the "native" form of the *IDH* gene is related to de novo primary tumors. Immunostains for MGMT (Fig. 5.94), ATRX, TERT, BRAF, and p53 are also useful.

5.11.5 Oligodendroglioma

Cytologic samples show a finely granular and frequently mucoid background, sometimes with microcalcifications. Often a delicate branching "chicken-wire" capillary network is observed. The neoplastic cells have an ill-defined and wispy cytoplasm with few glial processes. The nuclei are

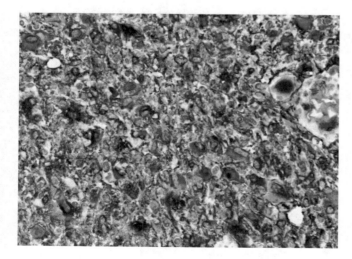

Fig. 5.91 Glioblastoma. GFAP immunostain (high magnification)

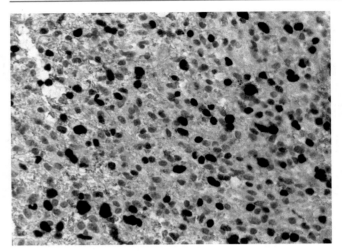

Fig. 5.94 Glioblastoma. MGMT immunostain (high magnification)

round with a crisp nuclear membrane, delicate "salt-and-pepper" chromatin, and small nucleoli. Oligodendroglioma shows loss of both the short arm of chromosome 1 (1p) and the long arm of chromosome 19 (19q); this co-deletion (1p/19q), together with the *IDH 1/2* gene mutation, is currently a mandatory requirement for the diagnosis. The conventional immunocytochemistry is positive for S-100 protein, galactocerebroside, carbonic anhydrase, CD57, and NSE.

5.11.6 Ependymoma

Cytologically, fragments of fibrillary tissue with discohesive sheets of relatively small cells are observed. In many cases, there are perivascular pseudo-rosettes, which have the characteristic "arboreal" or "caterpillar" features due to the fibrillary areas that separate the nuclei of the neoplastic cells from the walls of the vessels. The cells of ependymoma are uniform with a columnar-shaped cytoplasm, round to oval nuclei with granular "salt-and-pepper" chromatin, and inconspicuous or small nucleoli. The neoplastic cells are positive for GFAP, S-100 protein, NSE, podoplanin, NeuN, and CD56. Some cells express synaptophysin, CD99, CK8, and CK18.

5.11.7 Central Neurocytoma

Cytologic preparations from the tumor show round, monomorphic cells with ill-defined cytoplasm, uniform nuclear size and shape, finely stippled granular chromatin, and prominent nucleoli. The background is fibrillary. Tumor cells express synaptophysin, NeuN, and Hu.

5.11.8 Medulloblastoma

Cytologic samples of classic medulloblastoma are highly cellular and are composed of discohesive sheets of small, rounded or wedge-shaped cells with very scant cytoplasm. The nuclei exhibit folds and indentations and a slightly coarse "salt-and-pepper" chromatin without nucleoli. The desmoplastic/nodular variant exhibits an extensive finely granular background (neuropil matrix). The cytomorphology features are similar to those of the classic variant. The large-cell anaplastic variant shows large cells with large nuclei, coarse chromatin, and prominent nucleoli.

The neoplastic cells of the variants of medulloblastoma are variably positive for vimentin, synaptophysin, NSE, MAP-2, CD56, β-tubulin, and S-100 protein. Immunocytochemistry may be used for molecular classification of the tumor. Thus, the *WNT tumor type* shows *CTNNB1* and *APC* gene mutations and is positive for β-catenin, Yap-1, Otx2, and ALK. The *SHH-activated and P53-mutated tumor type* shows *TP53*, *PTCH1*, *SUFU*, and *SMO* gene mutations, and it is positive for p53, Yap-1, p75NGFR, and Gab1. The *SHH-activated and P53 wild-type tumor* has positivity for Yap-1, p75NGFR, NeuN, and Gab1. The *no-WNT no-SHH tumor group 3* has *MYC* amplifications and expresses Otx2 and PHOS, whereas the *no-WNT no-SHH type group 4* shows *MYCN* amplification and expresses only Otx2.

5.11.9 Meningioma

Cytologic samples exhibit polygonal (epithelial-like) or elongated (mesenchymal-like) cells or a mixture of these two cell types. The neoplastic cells have ill-defined cytoplasmic borders, slightly oval nuclei with delicate chromatin, and a single nucleolus (Fig. 5.95). Nuclear pseudoinclusions, con-

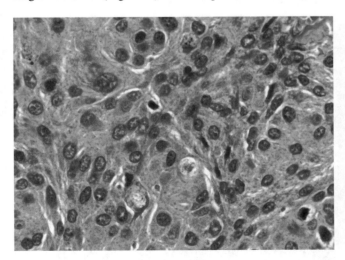

Fig. 5.95 Meningioma. H&E (high magnification)

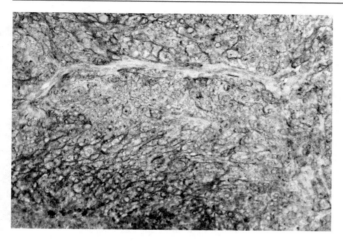

Fig. 5.96 Meningioma. D2-40 immunostain (high magnification)

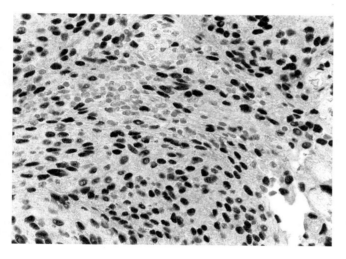

Fig. 5.97 Meningioma. PgR immunostain (high magnification)

sisting of invaginated cytoplasm pockets in the nuclei and clear "washed out" chromatin, are also present. The meningioma cells, independent of their shape, are positive for D2-20 (Fig. 5.96), E-cadherin, SSTR2a (somatostatin receptor 2a), vimentin, EMA, and PgR (Fig. 5.97).

5.11.10 Primary CNS Lymphomas

Various histotypes of primary lymphoma can be found in the CNS. The lymphoproliferative lesion that occurs most frequently is diffuse large B-cell lymphoma, whereas lymphoblastic lymphoma, Burkitt lymphoma, and anaplastic large-cell lymphoma are less common. The cytomorphologic features, flow cytometry expression, and immunocytochemistry of the primary CNS lymphomas are similar to those of lymphomas present in other organs. Therefore, please refer to the various paragraphs related to the cytology of lymphomas in this chapter and the previous one.

5.11.11 Metastases to the Central Nervous System

Numerous malignancies can involve the CNS by contiguity or by hematogenous dissemination. The cytomorphologic features and immunocytochemical characteristics of the metastatic deposit mainly reflect those of the primary tumor. In the case of a primary occult tumor, immunocytochemistry together with clinical data and imaging studies plays a decisive role in the identification of primary site.

Lung adenocarcinoma This shows papillary structures, three-dimensional groups (cell balls), intra- or extracellular mucin, and TTF-1-and/or napsin A-positive immunostaining.

Squamous cell carcinoma Metastases may be recognized by the presence of broad sheets of cells and whorls. Immunocytochemistry cannot suggest the site of the primary tumor.

Small-cell (neuroendocrine) carcinoma This shows small cells, an inconspicuous cytoplasm, nuclear molding, stippled chromatin, and neuroendocrine marker positivity.

Breast carcinoma Metastases may show various cytologic patterns, but usually the cells have cytoplasmic vacuoles containing mucin and express GATA-3 and mammaglobin.

Clear-cell renal cell carcinoma This often displays sheets of large cells with clear "foamy" cytoplasm, prominent nucleoli, and positivity for PAX-2 and PAX-8.

Urothelial cell carcinoma Metastases show flattened sheets of cells with homogeneous cytoplasm, a blunt pole that contains the nucleus, and positivity for GATA-3 and p63.

Colonic carcinoma This usually has columnar cells that express CK20 and CDX-2.

Melanoma Metastases show cell pleomorphism, as well as positive immunostaining with Melan-A and HMB-45.

Suggesting Reading

Baek HW, et al. Diagnostic accuracy of endoscopic ultrasound-guided fine needle aspiration cytology of pancreatic lesions. J Pathol Transl Med. 2015;49:52.

Bardales RH. Cytology of the mediastinum and gut via endoscopic ultrasound-guided aspiration. Cham: Springer International Publishing; 2015.

Cavallaro G, et al. Duodenal gastrointestinal stromal tumors: review on clinical and surgical aspects. Int J Surg. 2012;10:463.

Gimeno-García AZ, et al. Endoscopic ultrasound-guided fine needle aspiration cytology and biopsy in the evaluation of lymphoma. Endosc Ultrasound. 2012;1:17.

Hall BJ, et al. Fine-needle aspiration cytology for the diagnosis of metastatic melanoma: systematic review and meta-analysis. Am J Clin Pathol. 2013;140:635.

Kalhan S. Evaluation of precision of guidance techniques in image guided fine needle aspiration cytology of thoracic mass lesions. J Cytol. 2012;29:6.

Lacruz CR, et al. Central nervous system intraoperative cytopathology. Cham: Springer Science & Business Media; 2013.

Mathew EP, Nair V. Role of cell block in cytopathologic evaluation of image-guided fine needle aspiration cytology. J Cytol. 2017;34:133.

Sumana BS, Muniyappa B. Ultrasonography guided fine needle aspiration cytology with preparation of cell blocks in the diagnosis of intra-abdominal masses. J Clin Diagn Res. 2015;9:8.

Velez-Torres J, et al. Adult renal neoplasms: cytology, immunohistochemistry, and cytogenetic characteristics. Surg Pathol Clin. 2018;11:611.

Vilmann P, et al. Transesophageal endoscopic ultrasound-guided fine-needle aspiration (EUS-FNA) and endobronchial ultrasound-guided transbronchial needle aspiration (EBUS-TBNA) biopsy: a combined approach in the evaluation of mediastinal lesions. Endoscopy. 2005;37:833.

Vinayakamurthy S, et al. Role of cell block in guided FNAC of abdominal masses. J Clin Diagn Res. 2016;10:1.

Yang CS, et al. Percutaneous biopsy of the renal mass: FNA or core needle biopsy? Cancer Cytopathol. 2017;125:407.

Zhang R, et al. Combined endobronchial and endoscopic ultrasound-guided fine needle aspiration for mediastinal lymph node staging of lung cancer: a meta-analysis. Eur J Cancer. 2013;49:1860.

Pitfalls in Immunocytochemistry

6

It is important to have knowledge of the methodologies used in immunocytochemistry and to recognize the problems that cause procedural and interpretative errors in immunocytologic diagnosis. Lack of awareness of the pitfalls in immunocytochemical diagnostics can lead to potentially serious errors in diagnosis, which then affect patient management. This chapter covers in detail the causes of and solutions for these pitfalls.

6.1 Technical Artifacts and False Immunoreactions

The results of immunocytochemistry procedures and stains should not be considered as the results of activities that are independent of other "pre-analytical factors" to which the procedures are connected. Stain results are influenced by pre-analytic variables related to the preparation method used for the cytology sample, including sample fixation, antigen recovery, and eventual paraffin inclusion.

6.1.1 Artifacts Caused by Cytologic Sampling

Collection method The cell-sample quality influences the immunostaining. Cytologic sample collection maneuvers can result in inadequately collected cells, especially when the scraping method is used; cells can undergo cytoplasmic coagulation changes due to excessive heat caused by rubbing. The alterations which cells undergo result in morphologic changes (stretching and crushing), but the changes at the molecular level are much more important. In fact, cellular coagulation can provoke the migration and interstitial diffusion of oxidative enzymes, mainly lysosomal ones, which often produce diffuse non-specific immunostaining. Even cells that have undergone crushing or stretching trauma during collection frequently show a non-specific staining, regardless of the antibody used for the immunocytochemical

reaction, due to the diffusion of cytoplasmic and/or nuclear antigens into the extracellular space (Figs. 6.1 and 6.2).

Transport and prompt arrival The cytologic sample must arrive at the cytopathology laboratory not having been dried

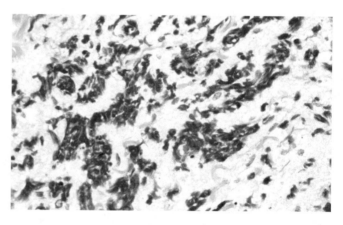
Fig. 6.1 Crushing artifact. H&E (high magnification)

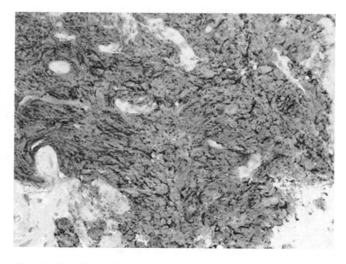
Fig. 6.2 Crushing artifact. Immunostain (high magnification)

and with viable cells. Furthermore, the cells must maintain their preserved antigenic structure unchanged; i.e., the classic canons of antigenicity must be respected: insolubility, accessibility, and preservation of the antigen. Cytologic material should be treated with fixative solutions or placed in transport medium immediately after sampling, to avoid cell drying, which causes modification of the electric charges and, therefore, favors the formation of non-specific bonds with the antibodies (Figs. 6.3 and 6.4).

Cellular ischemia Delay in the processing of fresh material causes the degradation of protein molecules, RNA, and DNA, as well as the activation of tissue enzymes and autolysis. Therefore, ischemia is a crucial factor influencing immunocytochemical results. Some antigenic molecules are particularly sensitive to ischemia; these include the majority of hormonal receptors, growth factors and their receptors, the molecules connected to cell proliferation, and phosphoproteins.

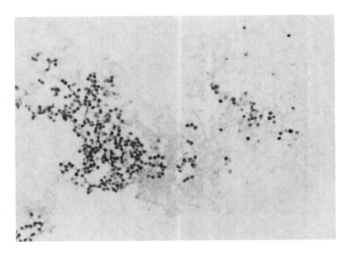

Fig. 6.3 Dried specimen. H&E (high magnification)

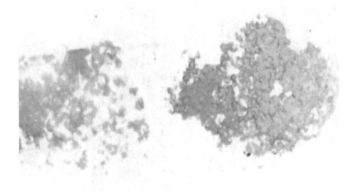

Fig. 6.4 Dried specimen. Immunostain (high magnification)

6.1.2　Selection of Cytologic Material for Immunocytochemistry

Sample adequacy The cytologic material to be used for immunocytochemical investigations must be adequate not only in overall cellularity, but also in an adequate number of elements that are representative of the lesion.

The problem concerning scarcity of abnormal cells in a cytology sample and subsequent immunostaining should be considered. If rare cells with cytomorphologic abnormalities are present, a single atypical cell showing positive immunostaining may be sufficient to suggest the diagnosis. On the contrary, negative immunostaining in the absence of atypical cells should be considered inadequate for diagnosis. In the event that the cytologic specimen was prepared only by smears, immunostaining should be performed on preparations harvested from different areas of the same specimen. However, if the number of smears is limited, immunostaining can be performed on Papanicolaou- or H&E-stained material after photographing/scanning of the cytologic preparation for archival purposes. If it is necessary to perform more than one immunostaining and the number of smears is small, another possibility is that of dividing the cytologic smear into two or more parts, delimiting the areas of interest by means of an "isolating pen" (Fig. 6.5). This method is particularly applicable to thin-layer preparations (Fig. 6.6). Furthermore, it is also possible to carry out immunostaining for two different antibodies simultaneously on the same cytologic preparation (Fig. 6.7).

Non-diagnostic elements in the sample The cytologic sample must meet certain requirements: having little or absent blood, not containing abundant acute inflammation, and lacking fibrin clots. When an immunoperoxidase reaction is used on cytologic samples with an abundant hemorrhagic fibrinous component or on highly proteinaceous material, the smear background usually stains intensively and can interfere with the normal reading of the immunoreaction (Fig. 6.8). Therefore, in the case of bloody FNA samples, it is advisable to wash the sample with solutions, such as cytolite, Esposti's solution (used particularly in Europe), or similar solutions before setting up the cytologic preparations, or to use a strong solution to inhibit endogenous peroxidase (Fig. 6.9). A short post-fixation in formalin is also useful; this can contribute to the lysis of red cells and to the blockage of endogenous peroxidase.

Similarly, the presence of large quantities of granulocytes and the consequent release of lysosomal enzymes cause a marked increase in background noise if peroxidase is used as an immunocytochemical tracer. This phenomenon is attributable to the release of oxidative enzymes that produce changes

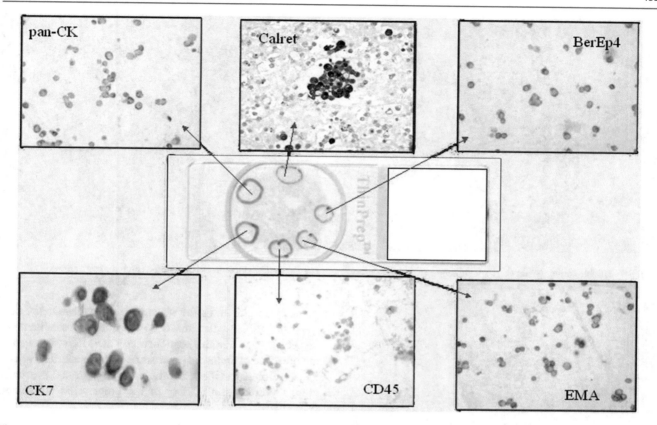

Fig. 6.5 Divided specimen on ThinPrep

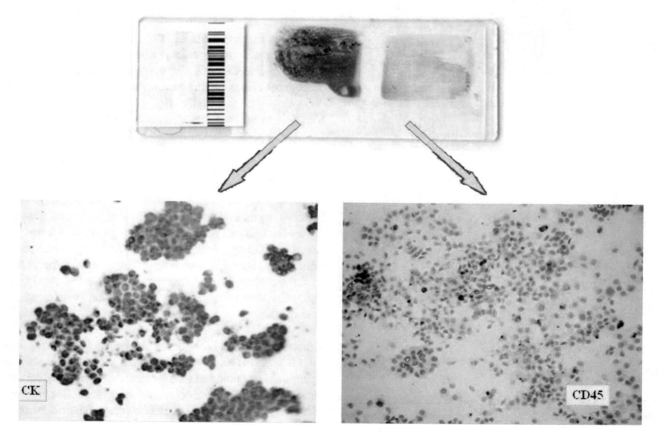

Fig. 6.6 Divided specimen on conventional smear

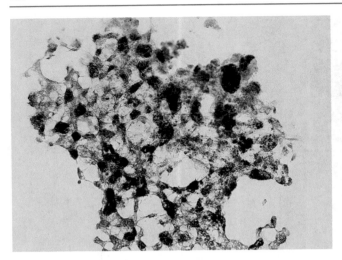

Fig. 6.7 Double immunostain (high magnification)

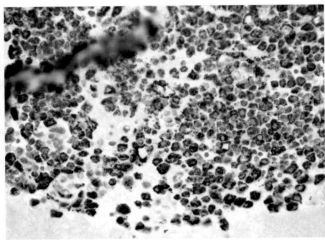

Fig. 6.10 Granulocyte-rich specimen (high magnification)

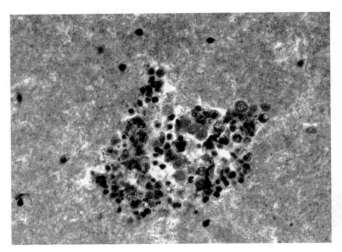

Fig. 6.8 Hematic specimen without peroxidase inhibition (high magnification)

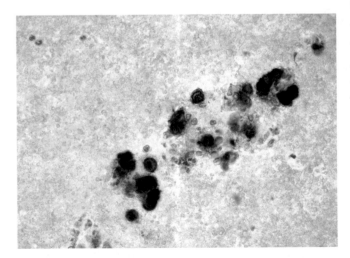

Fig. 6.9 Haematic specimen with peroxidase inhibition (high magnification)

in the molecular antigenic structure of the cells. On the contrary, the antigens that make up the intermediate filaments (especially cytokeratins) can maintain their integrity even in the presence of abundant necrosis or under conditions of cellular necrobiosis. Of course, the noise background is usually high; therefore, the reading of the preparation is difficult (Fig. 6.10).

6.1.3 Fixation and Fixative Solutions

Fixation is perhaps the most important parameter in the pre-analytical phase of immunocytochemical reactions, because inadequate selection of fixative solutions, times, and fixation procedures causes important variations in immunostaining.

Fixation time Inappropriate fixation can partially destroy the antigenic determinants or alter their structure until they are no longer recognizable by the antibody. An unfixed antigen can disappear completely or spread from the synthesis site into the surrounding tissue. Diffusion of the intracellular antigens may also be the result of a prolonged interval between the time of collection of the sample and its fixation. Under-fixation can preserve the antigen but can damage the tissue morphology, with consequent difficulty in interpretation. On the contrary, with longer fixation times, the quality of the morphology may improve, but a greater quantity of antigenic determinants may be masked, denatured, or destroyed.

Ethanol (ethyl alcohol) This is the typical coagulating fixative. It removes water molecules and therefore destabilizes hydrophobic bonding of the proteins, deploying their tertiary structure with the final outcome of protein denaturizing. Ethanol fixation does not affect all antigens, but most hematolymphoid markers and some antigens, particularly those rich in carbohydrates, may be deprived of their antigenicity. Destruction of the mitochondria, the structures of the Golgi apparatus, and the membranes of the secretion granules is observed. The antigenicity is modified in molecules that are rich in lipids and glycols, whereas it is preserved only for structures such as the intermediate filaments of the cytoskeleton and for some enzymatic activities. We have demonstrated that hyper-fixation in absolute ethyl alcohol favors the non-specific immunocytochemical marking of the nucleus. Moreover, inadequate preservation of some cell growth factor peptides and a possible shift in intracellular immunoreactivity has been observed; therefore, immunostainings will be falsely negative when hyper-fixation with ethyl alcohol is used.

Formalin   Cytologic material including cell blocks and, in some cases, smears can be fixed in neutral formalin-buffered solutions (see Chap. 1). The antigenic structures are usually preserved in their basic amino acid composition, but they are often "hidden" by cross-linking between the formalin and proteins. The proteins therefore undergo a certain denaturation, with partial disruption of secondary structures and tertiary complexes. This phenomenon is greater when the fixative is old and/or when the sample remains in the formalin-fixing solution for a long time. In this case, possible over-fixation artifacts must also be considered. The cross-links between the formalin and the active groups of proteins often prevent the recognition of amino acid sequences by antibodies and, therefore, cause the inevitable reduction or absence of the immune complex formation, and they reduce or abolish the immunocytochemistry staining. Formalin does not dissolve the lipids that are fixed through oxidation processes; however, fixing of glycols is practically impossible because these are found in aqueous solution and are therefore dissolved when formalin is used. Excessive fixation can cause irreversible damage to some epitopes, especially for nuclear antigens and markers related to cell proliferation, such as MIB-1.

An evaluation of the preservation of the antigen can be carried out by immunostaining with vimentin, an intermediate filament sensitive to fixation, which is typically expressed by vascular- or connective tissue cells. This immunostaining is therefore an internal indicator (control) of the preservation or loss of antigenicity.

6.1.4   Antigen Retrieval

If the antigen is masked due to cross-linking phenomena induced by the fixative, some procedures can be used for restoring the native molecule. The restoration of lost antigenicity must always be carried out in the event of fixation with formalin or with other fixative solutions that have the same mechanism of action.

There are different procedures for restoring antigenicity, which, however, are not equivalent to each other. It is therefore necessary to choose, among the various methods that are available, the most suitable one for use in relation to the type of antigen to be restored and the type of cytologic preparation. Whichever system is selected, the procedures should neither adversely affect the morphology of the individual cells or tissue fragments, nor should they intervene negatively by increasing the background of immunocytochemical stains. In the case of sections obtained from cell blocks, the antigenic reactivation can also be performed in the context of procedures carried out with fully automatic immunostainers.

The application of procedures for the recovery of epitopes in cytologic preparations not fixed with solutions containing aldehydes, theoretically, should be without effect because no molecular bridges have been created between cell antigens and the fixative. In reality, it is observed that the execution of a mild antigen reactivation treatment improves the immunostaining performance for a certain number of antigens. Unfortunately, the use of fully automatic equipment does not allow the execution of mild reactivating procedures. In the case of cell-block sections, the execution of an antigenic recovery procedure that is too mild does not allow for the complete recovery of the molecular structure of the antigen; therefore, the result is often a false-negative immunostaining (Figs. 6.11 and 6.12).

Time and temperature effect   The antigenic reactivations performed for too-long times or with too-high temperatures can destroy the antigenicity and alter the cytomorphologic aspect of the cells. High temperatures can cause lipofuscin artifacts. Furthermore, long antigenic restoration treatments at high temperatures can drastically modify the molecules and therefore create chimeric antigens (Fig. 6.13). In this case, the immunostaining may be either false-positive or

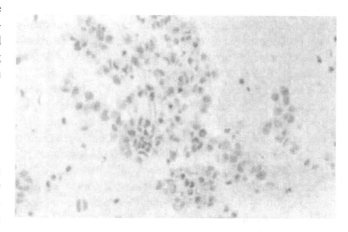

Fig. 6.11 Cell-block section without antigen retrieval (high magnification)

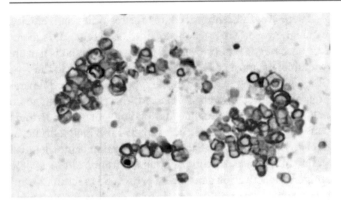

Fig. 6.12 Cell-block section with antigen retrieval (high magnification)

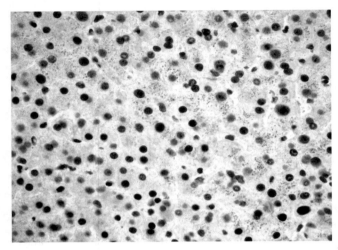

Fig. 6.13 Nuclear artifact due to antigen retrieval (high magnification)

false-negative. If too-high temperatures have been used, it is possible to identify the "burn" morphologic pattern in the adjacent loose connective tissue and fat.

Buffer effect The type of buffer solution used for antigenic reactivation, its molarity, and its pH can also significantly affect immunostaining. Some antigens are reactivated at acid pH, whereas others are restored only with the use of buffers having a basic pH. Many antigens do not show obvious differences with the use of citrate buffer at pH values between 4.0 and 10.0, whereas other molecules, in particular the Mib-1 and hormonal receptors, undergo a sharp decrease in their antigenic recovery when solutions with pH between 3.0 and 6.0 are used (Figs. 6.14 and 6.15). EDTA-based reactivating solutions often offer better results than does citrate buffer in antigenic recovery, although they must be used more carefully. Non-specific bonds between the antibody and some nuclear proteins can be observed after the use of buffer solutions of zinc sulfate, citrate at pH 6.0, and Tris at pH 9.0.

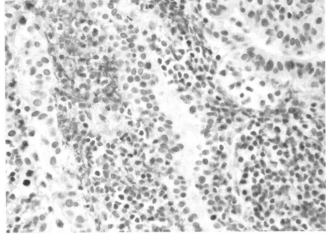

Fig. 6.14 Poor antigen recover due to inadequate pH (high magnification)

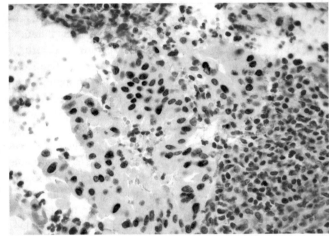

Fig. 6.15 Correct antigen recover by adequate pH (high magnification)

6.1.5 Endogenous Enzyme Blocking

In the performance of immunocytochemical reactions, enzymatic tracers (peroxidase and/or alkaline phosphatase) are used for detection of the result of immunostaining. Therefore, it is essential to use blocking systems for the possible endogenous presence of these enzymes, which produce an immunocytochemical stain that cannot be differentiated from that produced by the enzymatic tracer. The fixation and processing procedures for biological samples reduce the enzymatic activities, but do not determine their complete elimination. Inadequate blocking of endogenous enzymes produces false-positive results of immunoperoxidase and immunophosphatase alkaline reactions.

Special attention must be paid to bloody samples, as they are rich in hematin, and to situations of a high presence of granulocytes and histiocytes, due to the presence of large quantities of cytoplasmic enzymes. In these cases, it is advisable to use strong inhibitors in order to suppress the endogenous peroxidase and avoid a false-positive immunostaining result.

Strong oxidants, such as hydrogen peroxide and periodic acid, must be used with caution and in low concentration for the inhibition of endogenous peroxidase, particularly for evaluating some membrane markers, such as CD4, which they oxidize and denature easily. Subsequent immunostaining may therefore be falsely negative.

Similarly, endogenous alkaline phosphatase should be blocked with levamisole solution when an immunophosphatase reaction is performed.

6.1.6 Primary Antibody

Background stain Several artifacts can be traced directly or indirectly to the use of the primary antibody. Hydrophobic interactions and ionic attractions play a fundamental role in producing the link between the antigen and the antibody, but they can also generate an intense noise background. These non-specific interactions/attractions can be blocked by the use of preincubations with any protein that has no affinity for the antigenic target, such as normal serum, bovine serum, gelatin, or dry milk.

Antibody storage Inadequate storage of antibodies for a long time at temperatures above 25 °C can lead to the formation of immunoglobulin aggregates or polymers, favoring polymerization phenomena. This prevents the exposure of Fab immunoglobulin fragments and makes this site unavailable for binding with antigen, causing false-negative immunostaining. Likewise, immunoglobulin aggregation increases the rate of hydrophobicity, which increases the background color. This phenomenon appears in amplified form especially in the case of primary antibodies that are directly conjugated with a tracer.

Antibody concentration The concentration of the primary antibody also plays an important role in the formation of both false-positive and false-negative immunostaining. It is intuitive that a very strong antibody dilution can cause false-negative results. Inappropriately high antibody concentrations can cause two different types of artifact. A high antibody concentration favors the non-specific bonds of immunoglobulin through mechanisms other than the specific binding of the Fab fragment to the target epitope and causes a significant increase in background noise. Similarly, an increase in the concentration of the primary antibody can favor non-specific bonds (false positivity), especially with nuclear structures.

6.1.7 Detection System

The detection system (secondary antibodies and enzymatic tracer) can also be critical in producing false immunostaining. Here, the main cause of artifacts is the inadequate pH of the solution where the antibodies linked to the tracer are dispersed. This solution constitutes the microenvironment for the subsequent binding reaction between the primary antibody and the secondary antibody system. It should be kept in mind that each detection system requires specific buffers stabilized with appropriate enzyme tracer-related pH. The inadequate pH of the solution containing the detection system generally causes false-negative results because the enzyme tracer is unable to carry out its function.

Chromogen Artifacts attributable to the chromogen often depend on the buffered solution in which chromogens are dissolved. Granular precipitates can be formed when the composition of the diluting solution is not compatible with the chromogen. These precipitates are due to the inadequate concentration of salts or due to an inappropriate pH and are identified on the surface of the immunocytochemical preparation, obscuring the immunostaining and making it illegible (Fig. 6.16). An excess of chromogen in the diluent solution also causes granular aggregates, which tend to precipitate.

Chromogen incubation time Another source of artifacts is produced by the duration of the reaction time of the chromogen: if the incubation time is too long, preparations with an intense background are obtained, and, often, it is not possible to differentiate between a true reaction and a false-positive one. On the contrary, with a very short reaction time, it is not possible adequately to color the positive cells, which therefore are difficult to detect or even appear falsely negative.

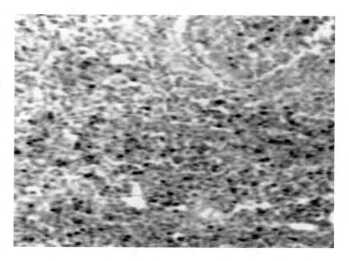

Fig. 6.16 Chromogen precipitates (high magnification)

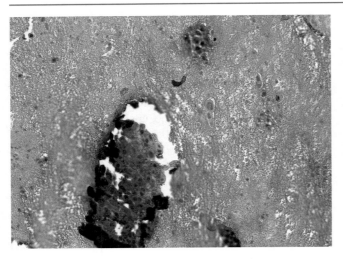

Fig. 6.17 Antibodies "trapping" (high magnification)

"Sequestration" artifact Another pitfall that occurs in the immunostaining of cytologic preparations is the so-called "sequestration" artifact of the reagent. This artifact can be seen both in cytologic smears, especially if the sample has conspicuous three-dimensional aggregates, and in cell-block preparations. This is a non-specific staining (false-positive) due to the precipitation of the chromogen, which remains trapped in the three-dimensional structures of the cytologic smear. A similar artifact occurs in cell-block preparations in areas of tissue section irregularity, distention of the sections, or by detachment of small fragments following antigenic recovery procedures (Fig. 6.17). These pitfalls are observed particularly when the sample has been insufficiently fixed, and sometimes in the presence of adipose tissue, and lead to consideration of the finding as positive.

6.1.8 Automated Immunostaining Artifacts

An important problem concerns the comparison of immunostaining performed manually to that carried out by an automated immunostainer. On the one hand, automation has significantly improved the reproducibility and reliability of immunocytochemical investigations, but on the other hand, it does not allow for optimization or flexibility in the use of reagents and antigen recovery methods. Therefore, the execution of immunocytochemical reactions on conventional cytologic smears and on thin-layer preparations is particularly difficult and sometimes impossible. Thus, there are advantages and disadvantages for both methods.

With fully automated immunostaining systems, it is possible to witness the formation of some artifacts; some errors are operator-dependent, and others are independent of the actions of the immunocytochemical staff.

"Open" and "closed" instruments Errors in programming of the procedure or in the imprecise positioning of the samples inside the instrument result in false stains. These artifacts are currently reduced considerably by the new instruments which, by use of direct reading and use of barcodes or analogues, of both the slide and the reagents, correctly match the samples with the reactions to be carried out. However, anomalies in the mechanical system and in the application of programs in the instrument can generate artifacts, regardless of whether the machine has an "open" or "closed" structure. One or more of the reagents required for immunostaining may be missing, with the consequent partial or total absence of immunostaining. A defect in the distribution of reagents can favor the formation of air bubbles on the slides, with consequent formation of circular areas without staining.

Evaporation of the reagent Another technical cause that can generate erroneous interpretation is the rapid evaporation of the reagents during incubation. This makes the cytologic preparation partially or entirely dry. The microscopic observation will therefore be of a monotonous immunostaining, or even the absence of immunostaining.

Slide-holder alignment Finally, another artifact may be observed when the plane of the slide holder in the instrument is not perfectly horizontal, and therefore the solutions delivered on its surface tend to flow, leaving the slide devoid of the reagents that are necessary for the immunostaining of the sample.

6.2 Pitfalls in the Interpretation of the Immunostains

It is important to realize that immunocytochemical reactions are not comparable to "special histochemical stainings," but rather are molecular investigation procedures, for the recognition of particular molecules present in cells whose identification allows one to refine the diagnosis or to direct specific therapies.

Many technical factors influence the immunocytochemical results, as referred to above. Negative, weak, or uninterpretable results should lead the pathologist to repeat immunostaining by using appropriate protocols and controls. But we must also consider any errors by the pathologist in the procedure selection and in the interpretation of the results. The interpretation of the results of immunocytochemical stains is best carried out by pathologists who have an adequate level of experience not only in the morphologic aspects of a diagnosis but also in immunohistochemistry and immunocytochemistry. Despite the best education, knowledge, and experience of the pathologist, errors of interpretation may occur.

6.2.1   Antibody Selection and Validation

The target molecule is identified through the use of antibodies that recognize one or few epitopes of the antigen. Therefore, different antibodies for the same target molecule can produce very different results. Thus, the correct choice of the procedure and of the antibody to be used is critical.

Monoclonal versus polyclonal antiserum   The selection of the antibody concerns primarily the choice between a monoclonal versus a polyclonal antiserum. As is known, the characteristics of these two reagents are different, and the choice of one or the other implies the knowledge of their differences and of their sensitivity and specificity. In fact, the monoclonal antiserum is composed of antibodies all of which are equal and are directed against the same epitope of the antigen molecule, whereas the polyclonal antiserum is made up of a mixture of antibodies that are different from each other and that are directed against the different antigenic determinants present on the antigen molecule. Therefore, it is necessary to use a monoclonal antibody to obtain greater specificity, whereas a polyclonal antibody is more suitable to meet the request for maximum sensitivity. For example, in the case of serous effusions, it is better to use a polyclonal antibody for CEA, as it is necessary to have the maximum sensitivity in the immunostaining of cells. In fact, about half of all adenocarcinomas are negative for monoclonal antibodies to CEA. The choice to use CD20 on cytologic samples of recurrent B-cell lymphomas of patients who had previous cancer therapy with monoclonal drugs leads to a diagnostic error with false-negative results (Fig. 6.18). In such cases, it is advisable to use the PAX-5 marker (Fig. 6.19).

Knowledge of the antibody   Wrong conclusions regarding the immunocytochemical picture can be made when the

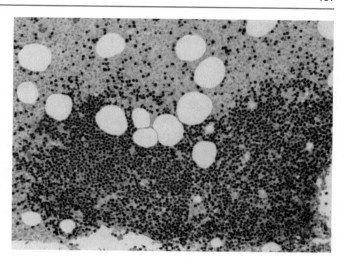

Fig. 6.19   Correct antibody (PAX-5) selection (high magnification)

knowledge about the characteristics of the antibodies is insufficient. One of the most common pitfalls is poor knowledge of the tissue and cellular distribution of antibodies directed against the so-called carbohydrate antigens (CA15.3, CA 19.9, CA 125, CA 150, and others). It must be remembered that these markers have a great aptitude for cross-reaction and that they react with several normal and neoplastic cells of different origins. Therefore, it is a mistake to consider, for example, CA125-positive cells as originating only in the ovary or CA15.3-positive cells as originating only in the breast.

6.2.2   Antigen Localization

The achievement of experience and adequate knowledge on immunocytochemical technology and its pitfalls, as well as the acquisition of specific and in-depth information on the biological characteristics of the antigens and on the specificity of the antibodies, prevent an incorrect diagnostic interpretation. The correct knowledge of the cellular distribution of a positive immunostaining that corresponds to the localization of the antigen (nucleus, cytoplasm, membrane, etc.) and the intensity and the type of staining (homogeneous, granular, point-like, and linear) obtained are the basis for a correct interpretation of the immunostaining.

"Unusual" antigen localization   It is also necessary and useful for diagnostics to have detailed knowledge that, sometimes, a seemingly abnormal immunolocalization of the antigen site in the neoplastic cell is not the result of an artifact but is the product of a true cross-reaction. For example, cytoplasmic immunostaining with TTF-1 antibody, exclusively the 8G7G3/1 clone, although resembling an artifact, is actually usable in the diagnosis of hepatocellular carcinoma; or

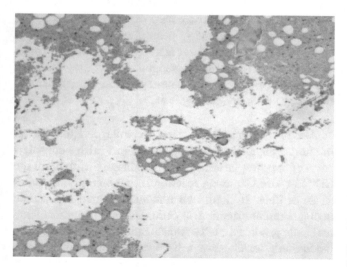

Fig. 6.18   Incorrect antibody (CD20) selection (high magnification)

the linear membrane immunostaining with Ki67 (MIB-1 clone) in a hyalinizing trabecular tumor of the thyroid supports its diagnosis.

Antigen migration A condition that can lead to considering immunostaining to be positive is the migration of the antigen from its normal location to another cell site or to the interstitium. This phenomenon is observed particularly during the immunohistochemical reactions for thyroglobulin, myoglobin, GFAP, and hormone receptors but can also occur with other protein molecules and is often due to a delay in specimen fixation. This positive immunostaining result must be known and not be interpreted in the context of cross-reactions. Non-specific interstitial staining can also be observed when a high concentration of serum immunoglobulins has abundantly permeated the sample before its fixation. To determine the real positivity, it is necessary to repeat the immunostaining on other samples.

6.2.3 Mistakes in Reading Immunostaining Results

An interpretative error can be avoided if the two fundamental parameters for the correct evaluation of the immunocytochemical results are kept in mind: the subcellular localization of the immunoreactivity and the type of immunostaining present.

Phagocytosis The phagocytosis of cellular micro-fragments by macrophages can constitute a pitfall in the reading of an immunocytochemical preparation because it is a false-positive reaction that looks like a real one. A similar finding of false positivity is due to the phenomenon of cellular cannibalism by neoplastic cells. The cannibalism of neoplastic cells does not always manifest by "eating" of cells or cell fragments; but sometimes cancer cells can only incorporate antigenic molecules from other cell lines: the result is, however, a false-positive one.

Cell damage During aspiration and extraction procedures, the cells can undergo crushing and/or stretching of the cytoplasm. These types of cellular damage cause the escape of cytoplasmic proteins that are arranged around the cell itself and cause non-specific bonds (false-positive) regardless of the type of antibody used for immunostaining.

Necrosis and apoptosis The individual cells harvested from infarcted or necrobiotic tissue result in nonviable elements present in the cytologic sample that can be a source of false immunostaining results (false-positive results), attributable in part to the release of cytoplasmic proteins and oxidative enzymes, which bind antibodies in a non-specific manner. Similarly, the immunocytochemistry of apoptotic cells and cells present in hemorrhagic areas can be interpreted mistakenly as positive due to the release of oxidative enzymes. Possible pitfalls, caused by the same phenomenon of non-specific bonds, can be observed in cells with abundant lysosomes rich in oxidative enzymes, such as those present in liver tissue and in granular cell tumors.

Mitochondria and RNA-rich cells Non-specific immunostaining, which can cause interpretive pitfalls, are also observed in cells with the presence of copious mitochondria, such as the oxyphilic cells of oncocytoma and Hurtle cell tumors. The cells of the granular layer of the epidermis, which are rich in RNA, can bind antibodies in a non-specific way, causing false-positive immunoreactions.

Edge of cell fragments Even the free edge of the sections obtained from a cell block, the external portion of the cell fragments in cytologic smears, and, sometimes, the cytoplasmic membranes of isolated cells can bind antibodies in a non-specific way, by electrostatic attraction causing false-positive images.

Pigment granules Pigment-laden macrophages or the pigment contained in other cell types can simulate a signal of immunocytochemical positivity, leading the inexperienced pathologist to false diagnostic conclusions. Among the pigments that can be misleading are the anthracotic, melanin, lipofuscin, and hemosiderin.

Interpretative errors: examples The observation of immunostaining of neoplastic lesions by inexperienced pathologists sometimes leads to the incorrect interpretation of a truly positive finding as false-positive or a technical artifact; such is the case for the expression of CK8 and sometimes CK18, in the presence of angiosarcoma, rhabdomyosarcoma, and leiomyosarcoma. In reality, the "aberrant" expression of cytokeratins in sarcoma cases is not a nonspecific stain or an artifact but is a true immunoreaction due to the synthesis of this molecule determined by a de-repression gene, as demonstrated by molecular biology tests.

Another example of incorrect interpretation of an immunocytochemical finding is determined by consideration of the cytoplasmic and/or membrane positivity of the CD246 (ALK) immune reaction in large-cell lymphomas as an artifact. It should be remembered that the classic nuclear immunostaining is observed only for the fusion molecule produced by the translocation t(2; 5). In molecular variants which always have involvement of chromosome 2, the antigen can be localized at the cytoplasmic or membrane level.

E-cadherin immunostaining is known to be positive in ductal carcinoma, whereas the cells of the lobular carcinomas, due to alterations of the corresponding gene, do not express this antigen. The absence of immunostaining for E-cadherin is due to silencing (repression) of the *CDH1* gene. Sometimes the gene is not repressed but has undergone a mutation and therefore determines the production of an abnormal protein. *CDH1* gene mutations generate different transcripts in relation to the site of the point mutation; consequently, the products also show anomalies that are directly related to the type of the mutation. The presence of granular cytoplasmic immunostaining represents the solubilization in the cytoplasm of the truncated protein, whereas focal or dot-like immunostaining is usually caused by anomalies of the protein in its cytoplasmic domain. Therefore, only the cells with linear membrane positivity for E-cadherin must be considered to be from breast ductal carcinoma; incorrect interpretation of the immunostaining results may impact patient management.

Rapid and superficial observation of immunostaining may also be a source of interpretative error. Immunostained specimens must be observed very carefully, especially when there is intense inflammation that can hide the presence of rare neoplastic cells (Figs. 6.20 and 6.21). Another pitfall that can lead to false diagnostic conclusions is the immunocoloration of cytologic smears that are rich in three-dimensional structures or tissue flaps, which can be false-positive due to non-specific adhesion of the antibodies, especially those of the detection system, or, on the contrary, they can be negative due to non-binding of immunoglobulin with the antigenic site.

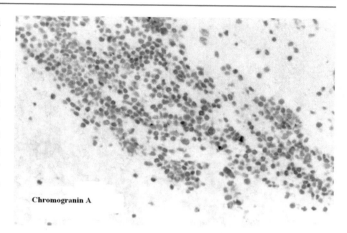

Fig. 6.21 Neoplastic cells hidden by inflammatory cells. Chromogranin A immunostain (high magnification)

Suggesting Reading

Bauer DR, et al. A new paradigm for tissue diagnostics: tools and techniques to standardize tissue collection, transport, and fixation. Curr Pathobiol Rep. 2018;6:135.

Bussolati G, Leonardo E. Technical pitfalls potentially affecting diagnoses in immunohistochemistry. J Clin Pathol. 2008;61:1184.

Chavali P, et al. Utility of immunochemistry in cytology. J Cytol. 2016;33:71.

Fitzgibbons PL, et al. Principles of analytic validation of immunohistochemical assays. Arch Pathol Lab Med. 2014;138:1432.

Fowler LJ, Lachar WA. Application of immunohistochemistry to cytology. Arch Pathol Lab Med. 2008;132:373.

Gown AM. Diagnostic immunohistochemistry: what can go wrong and how to prevent it? Arch Pathol Lab Med. 2016;140:893.

Kim S-W, et al. Immunohistochemistry for pathologists: protocols, pitfalls, and tips. J Pathol Transl Med. 2016;50:411.

Leonardo E, et al. Cell membrane reactivity of MIB-1 antibody to Ki67 in human tumors: fact or artifact? Appl Immunohistochem Mol Morphol. 2007;15:220.

Leong AS-Y. Pitfalls in diagnostic immunohistology. Adv Anat Pathol. 2004;11:86.

Libard S, et al. Characteristics of the tissue section that influence the staining outcome in immunohistochemistry. Histochem Cell Biol. 2019;151:91.

Lin F, Chen Z. Standardization of diagnostic immunohistochemistry. Literature review and Geisinger experience. Arch Pathol Lab Med. 2014;138:1564.

Miller RT. Avoiding pitfalls in diagnostic immunohistochemistry–important technical aspects that every pathologist should know. Sem Diagn Pathol. 2019;36:312.

Paavilainen L, et al. The impact of tissue fixatives on morphology and antibody-based protein profiling in tissues and cells. J Histochem Cytochem. 2010;58:237.

True LD. Quality control in molecular immunohistochemistry. Histochem Cell Biol. 2008;130:473.

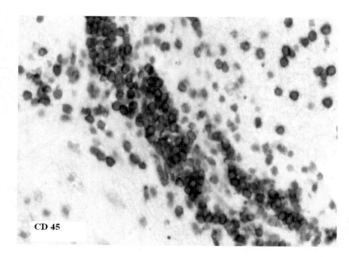

Fig. 6.20 Neoplastic cells hidden by inflammatory cells. CD45 immunostain (high magnification)

Index

© Springer Nature Switzerland AG 2020
E. Leonardo, R. H. Bardales, *Practical Immunocytochemistry in Diagnostic Cytology*,
https://doi.org/10.1007/978-3-030-46656-5

Printed in the United States
by Baker & Taylor Publisher Services